Multiple Sclerosis in Clinical Practice

Multiple Sclerosis in Clinical Practice

by

Aaron E. Miller MD

Division of Neurology
Maimonides Medical Center
Brooklyn NY
USA

Fred D. Lublin MD

Mt Sinai School of Medicine
Neurology Department
New York NY
USA

Patricia K. Coyle MD

Department of Neurology
SUNY at Stony Brook
Stony Brook NY
USA

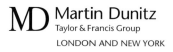

Martin Dunitz
Taylor & Francis Group

LONDON AND NEW YORK

© 2003 Martin Dunitz, an imprint of the Taylor & Francis Group

First published in the United Kingdom in 2003
by Martin Dunitz, an imprint of the Taylor and Francis Group, 11 New Fetter Lane, London EC4P 4EE

Tel.:   +44 (0) 20 7583 9855
Fax.:   +44 (0) 20 7842 2298
E-mail: info@dunitz.co.uk
Website: http://www.dunitz.co.uk

Although every effort has been made to ensure that all owners of copyright material have been acknowledged in this publication, we would be glad to acknowledge in subsequent reprints or editions any omissions brought to our attention.

The Authors have asserted their rights under the Copyright, Designs and Patents Act 1988 to be identified as the Authors of this Work.

Although every effort has been made to ensure that drug doses and other information are presented accurately in this publication, the ultimate responsibility rests with the prescribing physician. Neither the publishers nor the authors can be held responsible for errors or for any consequences arising from the use of information contained herein. For detailed prescribing information or instructions on the use of any product or procedure discussed herein, please consult the prescribing information or instructional material issued by the manufacturer.

A CIP record for this book is available from the British Library.

ISBN 1 901865 23 1

Distributed in the USA by
Fulfilment Center
Taylor & Francis
10650 Tobben Drive
Independence, KY 41051, USA
Toll Free Tel.: +1 800 634 7064
E-mail: taylorandfrancis@thomsonlearning.com

Distributed in Canada by
Taylor & Francis
74 Rolark Drive
Scarborough, Ontario M1R 4G2, Canada
Toll Free Tel.: +1 877 226 2237
E-mail: tal_fran@istar.ca

Distributed in the rest of the world by
Thomson Publishing Services
Cheriton House
North Way
Andover, Hampshire SP10 5BE, UK
Tel.: +44 (0)1264 332424
E-mail: salesorder.tandf@thomsonpublishingservices.co.uk

Composition by Phoenix Photosetting, Chatham, UK

Printed and bound in Spain by Grafos SA

Contents

Preface

The past two decades have seen an explosion of knowledge about multiple sclerosis, culminating in the introduction of the first treatments that impact the disease course. Exciting advances in immunology have led to better understanding of the immunopathogenesis of the disease. Development and continued refinement of magnetic resonance imaging techniques have led not only to improved diagnosis, but also to a dramatic increase in our understanding of the dynamic biology of MS. A steadily advancing science of clinical trial design and implementation has allowed the introduction, with Food and Drug Administration approval, of five medications that improve the disease course of MS into the United States market in the past 10 years. These include three preparations of interferonβ, glatiramer acetate, and mitoxantrone.

These substantial developments are often perplexing for the clinician dealing with the MS patient. Therefore, in this volume the authors have aimed to provide practical information that general neurologists, residents, primary care physicians and other health care professionals can readily use in helping them to better understand and care for their patients. Although each of the authors has a background and experience in laboratory neuroscience, they are primarily clinical MS neurologists who have cared for thousands of patients with the disease and participated in numerous clinical trials leading to the development of new treatments.

The volume begins with relatively brief chapters providing an historical context and fundamental background on pathology, pathogenesis, epidemiology, and genetics. However, the bulk of the text deals with practical clinical information concerning diagnosis, clinical features, imaging, and treatment. Extensive use of tables and illustrations should help provide a user-friendly approach to enable the reader to navigate the seas of this fascinating, but complex, disorder.

AEM
Dec 2002

Acknowledgments

I wish to acknowledge the contribution to my early understanding of MS by Dr. Labe C. Scheinberg, a pioneer in the modern, multidisciplinary care of MS patients. The late Dr. Murray Bornstein refused to believe there was not a treatment for MS and stimulated my interest in clinical trials. My greatest teachers have been my patients, without whom this book would never have existed. Linda Morgante, RN, CNS has shared my clinical work with MS patients for many years, during which she has taught me much about them and their care that I would not otherwise have understood. Most of all, I thank my wife Ellen and my daughters, Alexandra and Caroline, whose unwavering love and support have enabled my career and the writing of this book.

AEM

To Barbara, Alex and Derek for all their love and support
FDL

1
History

Although a relatively common neurological disease, multiple sclerosis nonetheless remains a mysterious ailment to much of the general public and, indeed, to many medical practitioners as well. A review of historic developments in the understanding of the illness and the management of those affected with it not only sheds light on current thought, but also provides insight into many of the medical trends of the last two centuries. For greater detail, the reader is referred to the thorough, scholarly review by Murray.[1]

Early cases

In the absence of any pathological confirmation or even contemporaneous knowledge of a disease process, it is, of course, extremely difficult to reliably assign a diagnosis, retrospectively, to any particular individual. Nonetheless, the description or writings of several persons strongly suggest the possibility, if not the certainty, of the condition.

The description of St Lidwina van Schiedam, who lived in the late fourteenth to early fifteenth centuries, is often cited as the first reported case. Her history was recounted in detail by Medaer[2] as follows (Figure 1.1):

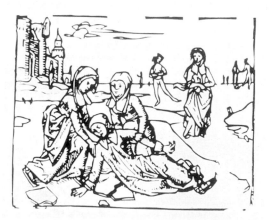

Figure 1.1
Woodcut illustrating St Lidwina van Schiedam whose history suggests she had multiple sclerosis. (Courtesy of Berlex)

Lidwina was born on 18 April 1380 in Schiedam, Holland. The years of her youth passed uneventfully. At the age of 12 she is described as being a healthy and charming young girl. In the following year she even received a proposal of marriage which she did not entertain.

On 2 February 1396, while skating, she fell and broke one of the right ribs. An abscess formed on the place of the fracture and the healing was difficult. The patient experienced walking difficulties and could move about only by seeking support on the furniture. There were also violent lancinating pains in the teeth (trigeminusneuralgy?) and headaches.

Several doctors were consulted, among them was one of the most famous, Godfried Sonderdank, court physician of Duke Albrecht of Holland and Duchess Margaretha of Burgundy. According to Brugman, he would have spoken to his colleagues as follows: "Believe me, there is no cure for this illness, it comes directly from God. Even Hippocrates and Gallenus would not be able to be of any help here. Let us admit this in all honesty rather than to bereave the poor father (Lidwina's) from his last means. The Lord's hand had touched this woman."

At the age of 19 walking became even more difficult and there appeared paresis of the right arm, as well as sporadic pains. Mention is also made of a split face and a hanging lip (fascialisparesis?). The right eye was blind while the left eye was rather oversensitive to light. Soon afterwards the patient is not able to walk and must be carried. There are also disturbances in the sensibility.

In 1413 appeared large wounds (decubitus?) for which Godfried Sonderdank was consulted again. With the assistance of a physician from Köln he succeeded in healing these wounds. There is some improvement in that the right arm became more mobile.

From 1407 onward a number of paranormal phenomena described as bilocation, contacts with God and the Angels, float over the bed.

Is it noteworthy that during these "extases" the patient should have a better sight and been able to move about easier (partial recoveries?).

During the following years there are progressively increasing swallow difficulties, at first with solid food and later on also with beverage. Fits of pains very similar to acute renal block are also described.

At the end of her life, she suffered from different wounds and she dies on 14 April, 1433.

St Lidwina's bones were recovered in 1947. Analysis did demonstrate changes consistent with paralysis of the legs, and probably of the right arm as well.

A very well documented case, before the disease was clearly recognized in medical circles, is that of Augustus d'Este (1794–1848) (Figure 1.2).[1] Augustus, the grandson of George III, kept a detailed diary beginning in 1822, in which he vividly recorded his symptoms and chronicled

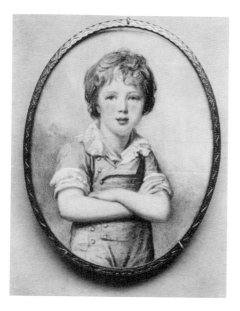

Figure 1.2
Augustus d'Este (1794–1848), here depicted as a child, kept a diary detailing symptoms of his disease which was almost certainly MS. (Courtesy of Dr. T. Jock Murray)

the progression of his illness over several decades (Figure 1.3). His initial account describes the development of blurred vision which progressed until he was unable to read. His vision subsequently cleared spontaneously, only to deteriorate again twice during the next few years. In the next few years he developed numbness in his legs and difficulty walking. He apparently recovered while receiving a variety of undoubtedly useless treatments which included the recommendation that he "eat beef steaks twice a day, drink London Porter and sherry and Madeira wines." Interestingly, he employed horseback riding as therapy, unknowingly anticipating the current equestrian therapy used by some MS patients, as well as those with other medical disabilities. He subsequently recounts symptoms suggestive of urinary tract infections, as well as difficulties with sexual function. Over the years, Augustus's diary recounts a host of encounters with prominent physicians and his trials with a variety of treatments, both physical and medicinal. By 1840, he had abandoned all therapy, apparently because of lack of success, but subsequently again tried various nostrums, including zinc sulfate, Spanish fly, strychnine, quinine, silver nitrate, and stramonium. His decline continued relentlessly, and his diary provides a glimpse into the practices of medicine and therapeutics available to the upper classes in the first half of the nineteenth century.

Another notable figure likely to have suffered from MS was the poet Heinrich Heine (1797–1856), whose work has been immortalized through the musical works of Schubert, Strauss, and Wagner.[1] As with the above cases, it is impossible to know with certainty whether Heine truly had MS.

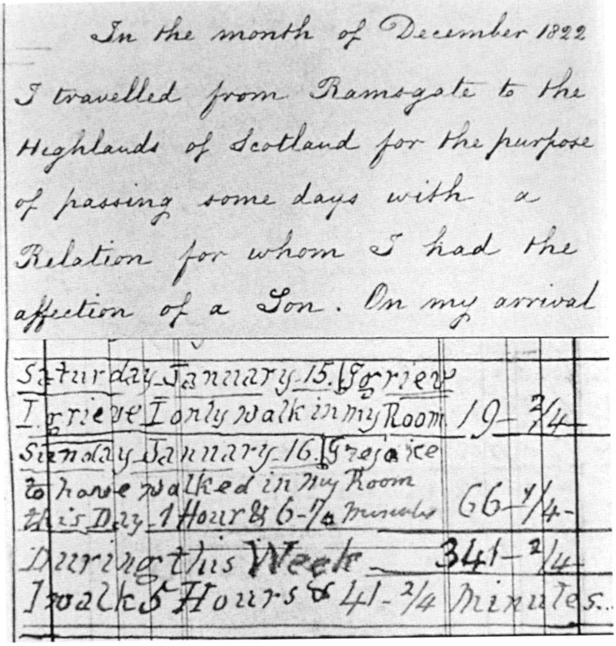
In the month of December 1822
I travelled from Ramsgate to the
Highlands of Scotland for the purpose
of passing some days with a
Relation for whom I had the
affection of a Son. On my arrival

Saturday January 15. I grieve
I only walk in my Room 19 – 3/4
Sunday January 16. I rejoice
to have walked in my Room
this Day 1 Hour & 6-3/4 minutes 66 – 1/4 -
During this Week 341 – 2/4
I walk 5 Hours & 41-2/4 minutes.

Figure 1.3
Handwriting samples from the diaires of Augustus d'Este. Note the deterioration as his disease progressed.

However, his illness was marked initially by transient weakness of the hands, followed by visual impairment which remitted only to worsen later, bulbar signs, and eventually progressive ataxic paraplegia – features strongly supportive of the diagnosis.

Early medical reports[1]

Charles Prosper Ollivier d'Angers probably provided the first report of MS in the medical literature in a monograph he published in Paris in 1824 on disorders of the spinal cord.[3] In his volume entitled "Maladies de la moelle epiniére", he described a 20-year-old man with relapsing-remitting neurological symptoms. He also provided the first description of the "hot bath test," reporting that his patient worsened when exposed to hot spa waters.

Robert Carswell first described the pathological changes of MS in an atlas published in 1838. He included a drawing of the spinal cord, pons, and medulla entitled "Brown transparent discoloration without softening of the spinal chord[sic]." (Figure 1.4) At virtually the same time, in France, Jean Cruveilhier reported four cases under the heading "Diseases of the spinal cord", describing patchy gray degeneration throughout the nervous system. Although Charcot credited Cruveilhier as the first illustrator of MS,[4] Carswell's pictures actually appeared 3 years earlier.

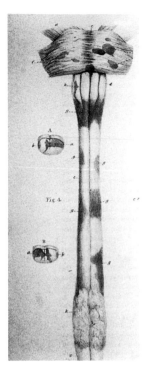

Figure 1.4
A drawing of the spinal cord by
Robert Carswell who first
described the pathology of MS in
1838. (Courtesy of Berlex)

Murray ascribes the first clinical diagnosis of MS in a living patient to the German clinician-pathologist Friedrich Theodore von Frerichs in 1849 (Figure 1.5). This case of myelitis was characterized by spontaneous remissions, and Frerichs further recognized the presence of nystagmus. Although critical comments followed Frerich's diagnosis, his student Valentiner subsequently published autopsy findings corroborating his mentor's impression.

The great French neurologist Jean-Martin Charcot (1825–1893) is undoubtedly the physician historically best associated with MS (Figure 1.6). Although neither the first to describe the disease clinically, nor pathologically, Charcot synthesized the features previously recognized by his colleague Edme Felix Alfred Vulpian, as well as his predecessors. Charcot's work defined the illness much more clearly and, perhaps most importantly, enabled other clinicians to recognize and begin to understand the condition (Figure 1.7).

In 1868 Charcot lectured the Société des Biologie on the characteristics of disseminated sclerosis (as the British would call it) and noted the distinctive clinical and pathological characteristics that allowed its differentiation from Parkinson's disease.[5] Later that year he published this lecture, as well as another report on the histopathology of the disease. Over the next few years Charcot studied additional and less severe cases and made

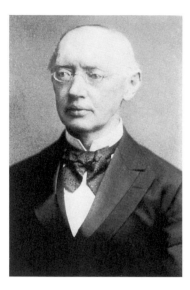

Figure 1.5
Friedrich Theodore von Frerichs, who made the first clinical diagnosis of multiple sclerosis. (Courtesy of Berlex)

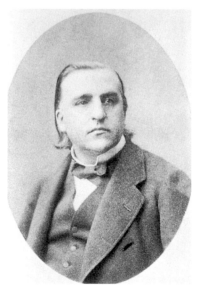

Figure 1.6
Jean-Martin Charcot, the French neurologist often credited with the most important early contributions to both the clinical and pathological understanding of multiple sclerosis. (Courtesy of Berlex)

many valuable observations, while always noting the contributions of others and emphasizing that he was adding further clarification to their work. Among the clinical features he observed were the transient nature of symptoms, the possibility of remissions, and variations in the clinical pattern of the disease. He recognized spinal, cephalic or bulbar, and mixed cerebrospinal forms. He described the tremor of MS; visual symptoms including nystagmus, diplopia, and amblyopia; speech disturbances; and intellectual impairment, including abnormalities of memory and concept formation. He also recognized the existence of pathological

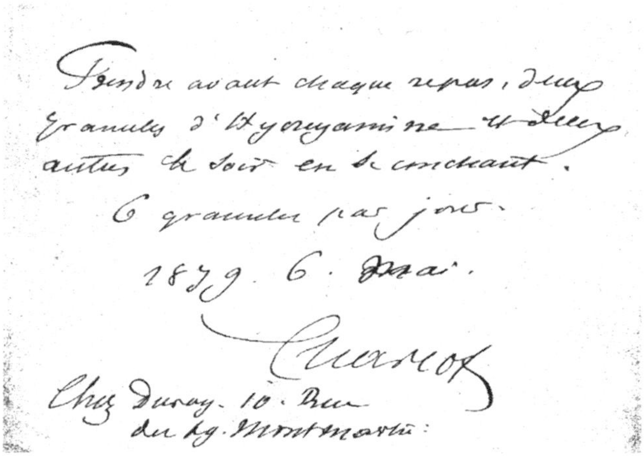

Figure 1.7
A prescription written
by Charcot. (From
the collection of
Barbara Lublin)

laughing and crying. He reported the characteristic combination of intention tremor, nystagmus, and scanning speech, ultimately eponymically
labeled Charcot's triad. Also a student of the pathology of the disease, the
French master identified myelin as the major target of attack. Although he
noted the relative preservation of axons, he was aware that they were
damaged at times.

Charcot's works became more widely known with the publication of his
Leçons in 1872–1873 and even further with their English translation published in 1877 in London and Philadelphia under the title, "Lectures on the
Diseases of the Nervous System."[6] Woodcuts from his classic 1868 paper
continued to be published well into the twentieth century (Figure 1.8).

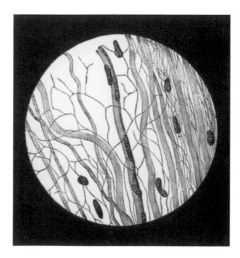

Figure 1.8
A pathological
illustration by Charcot.
(Courtesy of Dr. T.
Jock Murray)

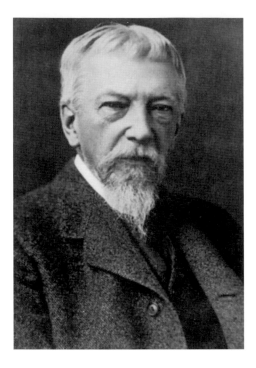

Figure 1.9
S. Weir Mitchell, famous American neurologist who provided a pathological description of MS in 1868, the same year as Charcot. (Courtesy of Berlex)

Although the brilliant contributions of Charcot have been widely acknowledged, he was not alone in his recognition of MS in that historic period. Across the Atlantic, in 1867 Dr J.C. Morris provided the first American report of a case.[7] This was published the following year – the same year as Charcot's original report – along with a pathological description by the famous American neurologist S. Weir Mitchell (Figure 1.9).[1] William Moxon provided the first major English language description with a report of eight cases, then called insular sclerosis, in the 1870s.[1,8] Noteworthy is his observation of the placebo response of MS patients, a phenomenon whose importance has been recognized in the recent plethora of major clinical trials.

First half of the twentieth century

The first half of the twentieth century witnessed little true progress in the understanding or treatment of MS. Searches for an infectious agent focused on the possibility of a spirochetal etiology, by analogy to syphilis. As the decades marched on consideration was also given to the possibility of a vascular etiology. Therapeutic efforts, uniformly unsuccessful or nonreproducible, followed the fashions of the day. Medication trials included antispirochetal agents, antihistamines, anticoagulants, and a variety of other agents. Equally ineffective were a variety of physical measures ranging from electrical stimulation to pelvic and rectal massage. The host of treatments attempted during this period are listed in Tables 1.1 and 1.2.

In 1933, Rivers, Sprint, and Berry reported the landmark development of the animal disease experimental autoimmune encephalomyelitis (EAE), which has served, albeit imperfectly, as a model of MS ever since.[9] The investigators initially produced an acute paralytic illness in monkeys by injecting homogenates of spinal cord in association with complete Freund's adjuvant. Because acute EAE is a monophasic illness, it does not faithfully mimic the course of MS. However, years later other scientists tweaked the immunization regimen in a variety of ways to produce models of chronic or relapsing EAE, first in guinea pigs and then in certain mouse strains[10-12] (Figure 1.10).

Intensive investigation of various EAE models has provided remarkable understanding of its immunopathogenesis. Insights gained from this work

Table 1.1 Treatments for MS before 1935

Treatment	Rationale*	Treatment	Rationale*	Treatment	Rationale*
Antimony	Inf	Gold chloride	Alt	Purves-Stewart vaccine	Inf
Anti-polio serum	Inf	Hydrotherapy	Phy, Psy	Quinine	Alt
Arsenic	Alt, Inf	Hypnotism	Psy	Salvarsan	Inf
Atoxyl	Inf	Kollargol	Uni	Silver nitrate	Alt
Autohemotherapy	Uni	Liver extract	Alt	Sodium salicylate	Ifl
Belladonna	Alt	Lumbar punctures	Phy	Solganol	Alt
Carbon arc	Phy	Mecury	Alt, Inf	Strychnine	Alt
Dental & tonsil extraction	Phy	Metallic salts	Alt	Tetrophan	Uni
Electrical stimulation	Phy	Neurosurgery	Phy	Thorium	Uni
Ergot	Alt	Nuclein	Uni	Ultraviolet	Phy
Fever therapy	Inf	Organ implant	Uni	X-ray	Ifl
Fibrolysin	Ifl	Potassium bromide	Alt	Zinc phosphate	Alt
Germanin	Inf	Potassium iodide	Alt	Zinc sulfate	Alt

*Rationales: Alt, "Alternatives"; Ifl. Anto-Inflammatory; Inf, Anti-Infectious; Phy, Physical; Psy, Psychiatric; Uni, Unidentified. (Courtesy of National Multiple Sclerosis Society)

Table 1.2 Treatments for MS from 1935 to 1950

Treatment	Rationale*	Treatment	Rationale*
Alcohol	V-D	Histamine iontophoresis	V-D
Allergens-desensitization	A-A	Neostigmine	C-S
Allergen-free diet	A-A	Niacin intramuscularly	V-D
Aminophylline	V-D	Papaverine	V-D
Amyl nitrite	V-D	Pelvic masage	Phy
Belladonna	V-D	Rectal massage	Phy
Caffeine	C-S	Syntropan	V-D
Deoxycorticosterone acetate (DOCA)	C-S	Spinal cord stimulation	Phy
Dicoumarol	A-C	Cyanocobalamin (Vitamin B12)	Vit
Ephedrine	C-S	Tocopherols (Vitamin E)	Vit
Etamon	V-D	Vitamins A, D, E and K	Vit
Histamine desensitization	A-A	Niacin	Vit
Histamine intravenously	V-D	Thiamin	Vit

*Rationales: A-A, Anti-allergic; A-C, Anti-coagulant; C-S, Circulatory stimulant; Phy, Physical; Vit, Vitamin(s); V-D, Vasodilating (Courtesy of National Multiple Sclerosis Society)

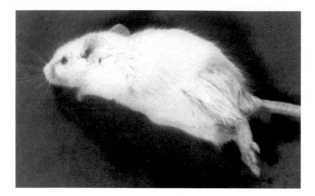

Figure 1.10
A mouse with severe experimental autoimmune encephalomyelitis (EAE). Note the paralyzed hind limbs. EAE is an often-used animal model for multiple sclerosis.

have been applied to MS and have led to the current view that it is an autoimmune disease of the central nervous system. Furthermore, EAE has served as a very useful testing ground for potential therapeutic modalities for MS. To be sure, many agents which have proved highly effective in ameliorating or preventing EAE have failed to benefit patients with MS. However, at least one currently approved treatment of MS, glatiramer acetate, owes its subsequent development entirely to early successful explorations in the animal disease.

The development of EAE, a noninfectious disorder, clearly representing an autoimmune phenomenon, did not preclude the possibility that a transmissible agent might play a role in the pathogenesis of MS. McAlpine's 1946 suggestion that MS is an immune reaction following an infection, setting up a potentially recurrent process, has recently been amplified by the concept of molecular mimicry.[13] This hypothesis postulates that an infectious agent shares antigenic determinants with a component of myelin, so that the immunological response to the pathogen is damaging to myelin.

Epidemiological and virological focus

As the twentieth century reached its midpoint and beyond, medical scientists increasingly recognized the importance of viral diseases and identified the specific pathogenic agents. At about the same time, particularly in the 1960s and 1970s, a series of epidemiological studies (detailed in Chapter 3) showed geographic variation in the prevalence of MS, with the disease occurring more often in temperate latitudes. Furthermore, a number of migrant studies suggested that the risk of the disease was acquired early in life. These observations dovetailed nicely with the possibility that the disease might be mediated by a particular viral infection during childhood. Enthusiastic embrace of this concept snowballed with the recognition of slow virus diseases, originally described by Sigurdsson in 1954.[14] In these disorders, initial viral infection is generally asymptomatic, but years later clinical manifestations develop. Sigurdsson's landmark paper detailed several slow viral infections in sheep, but soon thereafter human examples such as Creutzfeldt–Jakob disease (subsequently identified as one of a group of prion diseases), progressive multifocal leukoencephalopathy, and subacute sclerosing panencephalitis were recognized. The adult onset of MS combined with the migrant data suggesting early risk acquisition seemed a perfect scenario for the discovery of still another slow viral infection. Unfortunately, three decades later the quest for a specific pathogen remains unfulfilled.

The era of clinical trials

Treatment of MS remained unsuccessful and unscientific through the 1960s. Then, at the end of that politically turbulent decade, the groundbreaking trial of adrenocorticotrophic hormone (ACTH) for the treatment of acute exacerbations of MS, was led by Augustus Rose.[15] This represented the first successful randomized, double blind, placebo controlled multicenter trial in the disease and was the vanguard for the increasingly large and sophisticated clinical trials culminating in the development of new treatments in the 1990s. In this study, patients within 1 month of the onset of an acute attack were hospitalized and randomized to receive either 2 weeks of daily intramuscular ACTH or placebo injections and were followed to ascertain their rate and extent of recovery. The results demonstrated that patients receiving ACTH improved more rapidly, but ultimately no better, than those treated with placebo. This study also provides an interesting historic glimpse at changes in health care in the United States over the last 30 years. Imagine attempting to do a study today in which MS patients are hospitalized for 2 weeks to receive potentially sham intramuscular injections!

In order to conduct clinical trials, it is imperative to have agreement on the criteria used for diagnosis. Schumacher et al in 1965 provided the first widely used guidelines for this purpose (see Chapter 4).[16] Then, following the development of new electrophysiological techniques (evoked responses) and neuroimaging modalities, as well as increasing recognition of the utility of cerebrospinal fluid analysis, a committee chaired by Charles Poser proposed new and more complex criteria for the diagnosis of MS.[17] This scheme became the benchmark for diagnosis for the remainder of that decade, as well as the next.

Particularly during the 1980s the results of many trials employing a variety of immunosuppressive medications were reported. While many of these agents appeared to be beneficial during open-label or small randomized trials, most fell by the wayside or demonstrated only minimal effect when subjected to large, multicenter, randomized, double blind, placebo controlled studies. Despite the failure of these trials to identify effective therapeutic agents, they did serve as training ground for a cadre of investigators who became increasingly skilled in the conduct of these highly complex studies. These researchers, both in North America and Europe, were then primed to carry out the exciting trials in the 1990s of the interferons and glatiramer acetate (discussed in Chapter 7) which have led to regulatory approval of these agents, the first drugs clearly successful in altering the natural history of MS.

Nonprofit MS organizations

Another key development in the history of MS was the founding in the United States of the National MS Society (NMSS), originally called the Association for the Advancement of Research into MS, in 1945. The establishment of this organization resulted from the tireless efforts of Sylvia Lawry, who had been frustrated by her inability to find help for her brother who was suffering with the disease (Figure 1.11). This was followed by the establishment of the MS Society of Canada a few years later and then by similar organizations in other nations. The NMSS, as well as other MS societies, has been a mainstay of research funding for the disease, in addition to promoting improved care and advocacy for MS patients.

Following the pioneering efforts of Labe Scheinberg to develop a model of comprehensive care for MS patients, a number of such centers developed in the United States. In 1986, seven prominent MS centers founded the Consortium of MS Centers (CMSC) with a principal goal of improving the care of patients. This organization has since expanded to an international group with over 200 MS centers among its membership. An organization composed of a wide variety of professionals caring for MS patients, it has served as a forum for the exchange of information and a resource for the development of collegial relationships. The existence of the CMSC has undoubtedly contributed greatly to the expansion of the number of committed individuals working in the field, as well as to their retention in a very stressful professional area.

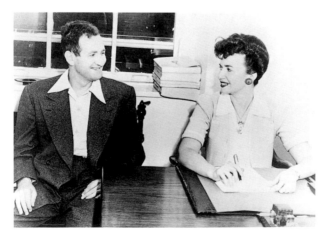

Figure 1.11
Sylvia Lawry (1915–2001) who founded the National Multiple Sclerosis Society (originally the Association for Advancement in Research into MS) in 1945 in an effort to help her brother who had been diagnosed with the disease. (Courtesy of National Multiple Sclerosis Society)

Summary

Progress in MS, since the pioneering work of Charcot and his predecessors, has occurred not by sudden, dramatic scientific breakthroughs, but through the continued efforts of thousands of investigators. Advances in understanding of basic science, particularly immunology, as well as developments in the investigation of clinical disease, especially magnetic resonance imaging, ultimately contributed to the approval of the first drugs to impact the natural history of the disease. At the dawn of the twenty-first

14th–15th century	St. Lidwina—possibly first described case suggestive of MS
1822	Augustus d'Este begins diary that chronicles his experiences with what is almost certainly MS
1824	Charles Prosper Ollivier d'Angers publishes first report of MS in medical literature
1838	Robert Carswell first describes pathological changes of MS
1849	Friedrich Theodore von Frerichs reports first clinical diagnosis of a living patient
1868	Jean-Martin Charcot gives first lectures to Societe des Biologie on the disease and goes on to describe many features of MS in his "Lectures on the Diseases of the Nervous System"
	J. C. Morris reports first American case
1933	Description of experimental allergic (autoimmune) encephalomyelitis by Rivers, Sprint, and Berry provides animal model of MS
1945	National Multiple Sclerosis Society founded in the US by Sylvia Lawry to promote research
1946	McAlpine suggests MS is an immune reaction following an infection
1960s–70s	Epidemiological studies demonstrate MS is more prevalent in temperate latitudes; migrant studies suggest an epidemiological factor is operative during childhood
1965	Schumacher provides first widely used diagnostic criteria
1970	Publication of first large randomized, double-blind, placebo-controlled trial in MS by Augustus Rose et al demonstrating that ACTH speeds recovery from an acute attack
1980s	Trials of many immunosuppressive agents for treatment of MS with marginal success
1983	Publication of new criteria for diagnosis of MS by committee chaired by Charles Poser
Mid 1980s	Introduction of MRI into clinical practice, leading to major advances in diagnosis
1986	Consortium of MS Centers founded, bringing a wide variety of professionals together, with the mission of promoting the care of MS patients
1993	Interferon beta-1b (Betaseron) becomes first drug approved for MS by the US Food and Drug Administration.
1996	Interferon beta-1a (Avonex) approved in the US
1997	Glatiramer acetate (Copaxone) approved in the US
2000	Mitoxantrone (Novantrone) becomes first drug approved in the US for progressive MS

Figure 1.12
Historical timeline.

century, the availability of the interferons and glatiramer acetate has accentuated the hopes of those afflicted with MS and their families and loved ones (Figure 1.12). If not the beginning of the end of MS, these treatments may at least mark the end of the beginning of the quest for the solution to this mysterious and often devastating disease.

References

1. Murray TJ. The history of multiple sclerosis. In: Burks JS, Johnson KP, eds. Multiple sclerosis: diagnosis, medical management, and rehabilitation. New York: Demos Medical Publishing, Inc., 2000: 1–32.

2. Medaer R. Does the history of multiple sclerosis go back as far as the 14th century? Acta Neurol Scand 1979; 60:189–192.

3. Ollivier CP. La Moelle Epiniére et de ses maladies. Paris: Crevot; 1824.

4. Cruveilhier J. Anatomie pathologicque du corps human, ou descriptions avec figures lithograpiés et coloriéts des diverse alterations morbides dout le corps humain est susceptibles. Paris: J.B. Ballière, 1835.

5. Charcot JM. Histologie de le sclérose en plaques. Gaz Hop Paris 1868; 554–558.

6. Charcot JM. Lectures on diseases of the nervous system. Translated by G. Sigerson. London: The New Sydenham Society. 1877.

7. Morris JC. Case of the late Dr CW Pennock. Am J Med Sci 1868; 56:138–144.

8. Moxon D. Case of insular sclerosis of brain and spinal cord. Lancet 1873; i:236.

9. Rivers TM, Sprint DH, Berry GP. Observations on attempts to produce acute disseminated encephalomyelitis in monkeys. J Exp Med 1933; 58:39–53.

10. Brown AM, McFarlin DE. Relapsing experimental allergic encephalomyelitis in the SJL/J mouse. Lab Invest 1981; 45:278–284.

11. Lassman H, Wisniewski HM. Chronic relapsing experimental allergic encephalomyelitis: clinicopathologic comparison with multiple sclerosis. Arch Neurol 1979; 36:490–497.

12. Lublin FD, Maurer PH, Berry RG, et al. Delayed, relapsing experimental allergic encephalomyelitis in mice. J Immunol 1981; 126:819–822.

13. McAlpine D. The problem of disseminated sclerosis. Brain 1946; 69:233–250.

14. Sigurdsson B. Observations on three slow infections of sheep. Br Vet J 1954; 110:255–270.

15. Rose AS, Kuzuma JW, Kurtzke JF, et al. Cooperative study in the evaluation of therapy in multiple sclerosis: ACTH vs. placebo. Final report. Neurology 1970; 20:1–59.

16. Schumacher GA, Beebe G, Kubler RF, et al. Problems of experimental trials of therapy in multiple sclerosis: report by the panel on the evaluation of experimental trials of therapy in multiple sclerosis. Ann NY Acad Sci 1965; 122:522–568.

17. Poser CM, Paty DW, Scheinberg L, et al. New diagnostic criteria for multiple sclerosis: guidelines for research protocols. Ann Neurol 1983; 13:227–231.

2
Pathology, pathogenesis, and pathophysiology

Pathology

The pathology of MS was first described in the 1830s by Carswell in London and Cruveilhier in Paris, well ahead of the subsequent clinical descriptions, best synthesized by Charcot, who also provided additional pathological detail. The early descriptions of MS pathology stressed the relative loss of myelin and preservation of the underlying axons. However, even the early descriptions noted that there was evidence for a degree of axonal damage (Charcot noted this in his early publications). In addition to the nerve fiber damage, another key element to the pathology of MS is inflammation. The inflammation is primarily perivenular, in the pattern of a cell-mediated immune response, and consists primarily of lymphocytes and macrophages. The MS plaque also demonstrates astrogliosis. In acute plaques there is evidence of active myelin damage (macrophages filled with myelin breakdown products) in association with perivenular inflammation (Figure 2.1). More recently, authors have stressed that the degree of axonal damage present, even in early lesions, can be considerable.(Figure 2.2)[1,2] As repair of axonal damage

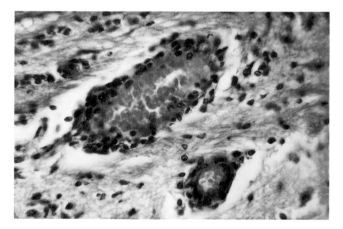

Figure 2.1
Petivascular infiltration of lymphocytes in an acute MS lesion.

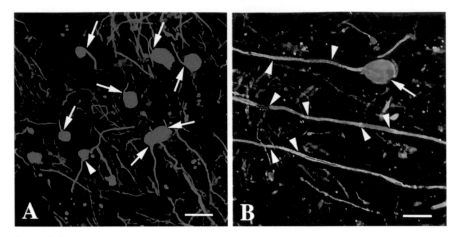

Figure 2.2
Confocal microscopic images of axonal damage in multiple sclerosis lesions.
Panel A depicts terminal axonal ovoids and Panel B shows concomitant acute
demyelination and axonal damage (From reference 1).

is less likely to occur than remyelination, the finding of early axonal damage
is of importance in developing treatment strategies, both in considering early
treatment and also for considering neuroprotective therapeutic approaches.
There is an important caveat in interpreting this data as it comes from autopsy
cases, which may represent a special subset of MS patients. The recent finding of MRI-measured atrophy early in the course of MS supports the concept
of important tissue loss, but as currently measured does not allow discrimination as to whether the tissue loss is due to myelin damage, axonal damage, or more likely, both. Further, in the acute lesion of MS, there can be
swelling that will increase brain volume. Treatment of this with anti-inflammatory agents will result in a reduction in brain volume and could be misinterpreted as atrophy using current MRI measures of brain volume. A full
segmentation analysis of the cerebral contents by MRI would allow improved
discrimination of the various compartments and structures, affording a
clearer understanding of the pathological consequences of both disease
progression and effects of therapy. MR spectroscopic changes in *N*-acety-
laspartate (NAA), a marker of neuronal function, have also been noted in
lesions of MS, supporting alteration of neuronal function in lesions at all
stages. Of interest, these changes are not always irreversible, suggesting
that NAA is a marker of neuronal dysfunction, not just destruction. In relatively
active, acute lesions oligodendrocytes are present, either spared or regen-
erated from a precursor pool. More chronic MS lesions have less inflammation, more astroglial scarring and a paucity of oligodendrocytes (Figure 2.3).
MS is a disease of the central nervous system (CNS), primarily, but not exclusively, of white matter. Recent MRI–neuropathological correlations have
demonstrated that lesions adjacent to cortical gray matter are common.

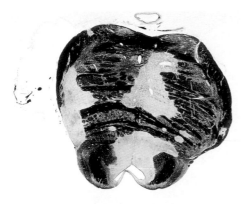

Figure 2.3
Section of the pons
stained for myelin
demonstrating
chronic patches of
demyelination.

A coordinated effort to better appreciate the pathological processes underlying MS has led to publication of a comprehensive classification of the pattern of acute demyelinative pathology seen in a sample of 51 biopsies and 32 autopsies.[3] The investigators were able to distinguish four patterns of demyelination in these specimens from MS patients (Table 2.1).

Patterns I and II were similar in that in both the active demyelination was associated with T cells and macrophages, usually in a perivenular distribution with the demyelinated areas showing sharply demarcated edges. There was loss of all myelin antigens simultaneously. There were remyelinated areas – shadow plaques (sharply demarcated lesions with thin

Table 2.1 Summary of pathological patterns and percentages

	Pattern			
	I	II	III	IV
T cells	+++	++	++	++
Macrophages	++	++	++	+++
Complement/IgG	–	++	–	–
Demyelination	Perivenous, sharp lesion edge	Perivenous, sharp lesion edge	Nonperivenous, ill defined lesion edge, concentric pattern	± Perivenous, sharp lesion edge
Oligodendrocyte loss	Variable	Variable	Pronounced	Pronounced
Oligodendrocyte apoptosis	–	–	++	–
Remyelination	++	++	–	–
Relative frequency	3	1	2	4

(Adapted from Lucchinetti et al.[3])

myelin sheaths throughout). Oligodendrocyte loss was variable at the active lesion borders and high numbers of oligodendrocytes in the inactive lesion center. In pattern II lesions there was prominent deposition of immunoglobulin and complement (specifically complement C9neo antigen).

In pattern III, there was inflammation with lymphocytes, macrophages and activated microglia. There was no deposition of immunoglobulin or complement. The demyelination was not perivenular. A rim of preserved myelin was frequently seen around inflamed vessels in the demyelinated lesion. The active lesions were ill defined, in contrast to types I and II. In several specimens, there were concentric alternating rings of demyelinated and myelinated regions at the periphery of the lesions. The most distinguishing feature of pattern III is the loss of myelin associated glycoprotein (MAG) while other myelin proteins (myelin basic protein, proteolipid protein, cyclic nucleotide phosphodiesterase) were still present in the damaged myelin sheaths. There was evidence of apoptosis of oligodendrocytes with loss of oligodendrocytes at the active lesion border and almost total absence of oligodendrocytes in the inactive centers of the plaques.

Pattern IV consisted of inflammation involving T cells and macrophages but no deposition of immunoglobulin or complement. There was demyelination and oligodendrocyte death at the plaque margins but no signs of apoptosis. There was equal loss of all myelin proteins in the demyelinated areas. There was extensive loss of oligodendrocytes in active and inactive lesions with no signs of remyelination.

The pattern most frequently observed was pattern II followed by patterns III, I and IV. Patterns I and II were common in cases of acute MS, but pattern II was uncommon in chronic MS. Pattern II was usually seen in patients with a short duration of disease. Pattern IV was uncommon, occurring in only three cases, all with a clinical pattern of primary progressive MS. Patterns I and II were seen in patients with all of the clinical course subtypes.

Of interest, in autopsy cases there was a tendency for all acute lesions to have the same pathological pattern, i.e., intrapatient homogeneity. These different patterns raise the possibility that MS may have different pathogenic mechanisms or etiologies and support the hypothesis of disease heterogeneity. This also raises therapeutic issues, as different inciting causes, and pathological patterns, may require different therapeutic approaches. The major caveat for this work is that it comes from autopsy cases, which provide only one time point for pathological assessment, and in most cases do not reflect early disease events. Biopsy cases represent, at best, very atypical presentations of MS, and thus may not represent the more usual pathological changes of the illness.

Pathogenesis

The underlying pathogenesis of MS is unclear as the cause of MS is unknown. The two currently favored hypotheses on the cause of MS are that it is either an autoimmune disorder or infectious disease, or a combination of both.

The basis for the autoimmune hypothesis comes from several lines of evidence, including the animal model experimental allergic encephalomyelitis (EAE), the nature of the pathological changes (described above), and the presence of a dysimmune state in patients with MS. The strongest evidence to date comes from the successful application of immunomodulating agents in MS, although the failure of immunosuppression, including bone marrow replacement strategies, speaks against an autoimmune hypothesis.

Experimental allergic encephalomyelitis (EAE) is a cell-mediated autoimmune disorder of the central nervous system (CNS) that has served both as a useful model of CNS inflammation, an animal model for MS, and as an easily evaluable and manipulable model for organ specific autoimmune diseases in general.[4,5] EAE is the most commonly employed animal model of MS, despite differences in the two conditions. The primary difference between these disorders is that EAE must be induced in animals, while MS occurs spontaneously in humans. There is no spontaneous occurring form of EAE in wild-type animals.

EAE, like MS, is an inflammatory, demyelinating disorder of the CNS, sparing the peripheral nerves. Both the clinical expression and pathological picture of EAE are similar to that seen in MS (Figures 2.4–2.6). As EAE is an autoimmune disorder, these similarities have provided strong evidence for MS also being an autoimmune disease. Similarly, as EAE is induced by specific myelin antigens, e.g., myelin basic protein (MBP) or proteolipid protein (PLP), attention in MS has focused on autoimmunity to these molecules. Both EAE and MS appear to be mediated by CD4+ T cells, are dependent on expression of the appropriate MHC class II (HLA,

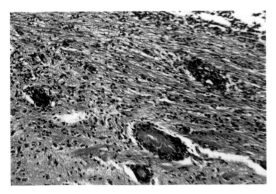

Figure 2.4

Perivascular lymphocytic infiltrate in the spinal cord of a mouse with EAE.

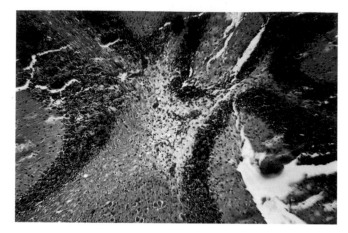

Figure 2.5
Area of chronic demyelination in the cerebellum of a mouse with relapsing EAE.

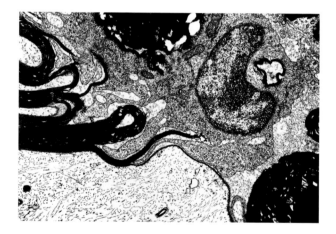

Figure 2.6
An electron micrograph of a macrophage in the act of peeling (phagocytosing) myelin from a nerve fiber (axon lower left). The macrophage is a monocyte from the peripheral blood and already contains large droplets of myelin debris. Cell processes from the macrophage can be seen separating the layers of myelin. Rabbit EAE at 7 months. Magnification ×15,000. (Courtesy of Dr Cedric Raine.)

Ia) antigens, specific T cell receptor bearing lymphocytes, adhesion molecule expression, and cytokine secretion. Both diseases are organ specific, affecting solely myelin from the CNS, and require trafficking of lymphocytes from the periphery across the blood–brain barrier (BBB) into the

CNS. New experimental and pathological data suggest that antibodies to CNS antigens may play a similar role in the pathogenesis of both EAE and MS, in addition to cell-mediated immune mechanisms[6] (Table 2.2).

The immune pathogenesis of MS centers on the T lymphocyte. T cells can be divided into CD4+ and CD8+ subsets.[7] CD4+ T cells mediate the encephalitogenic course of EAE. There is no clear role for CD8+ T cells in the immunopathogenesis of MS, although abnormalities of this subgroup have been described in MS patients. The CD4+ T cell subset can be further subdivided into T helper (Th) 1 and 2. Th1 cells mediate delayed type hypersensitivity reactions, such as EAE, and downregulate Th2 cells. Th2 cells are involved with antibody-mediated events and tend to antagonize the effects of Th1 cells. This contraregulation is due, at least in part, to the differential cytokine secretion patterns of these T cell subsets. Th1 cells secrete the proinflammatory cytokines (interleukin) (IL)-2, interferon (IFN) γ and tumor necrosis factor α (TNF-α, lymphotoxin). Th2 cells secrete IL-4, IL-5, and IL-10. IL-4 and IL-10 have inhibitory effects on Th1 cells. Myelin antigen reactive CD4+ T cells of the Th1 subtype mediate EAE, while those of the Th2 subtype usually do not. Further, treatment of MBP specific T cells with IL-4 can transform T cell populations from Th1 to Th2 and ameliorate the effects of EAE. The EAE model has provided the best evidence for use of immune deviation techniques in the treatment of autoimmune demyelination. The logic of immune deviation involves a switch from a Th1 predominant immune response to a Th2 response, with the attendant switch in cytokine secretion from immune enhancing to immunosuppressive. This approach is thought to underlie the use of oral antigen and altered peptide ligand (APL), neither of which has been a very promising approach in initial

Table 2.2 Comparison of features of EAE and MS.

	EAE	MS
CNS signs	+++	+++
Relapsing disease	++	+++
CNS perivascular inflammation	+++	+++
CNS demyelination	+ → +++	+++
Antibody-mediated demyelination	++	++
CNS remyelination	++	++
Oligodendrocyte loss	–	+ → +++
Immunogen	MBP, PLP, Myelin Oligodendrocyte Glycoprotein, others	Unknown
Genetic predisposition	++	++
Linked to MHC	++	++
Limited T cell receptor heterogeneity	+	+
Microbial precipitant	+	++
Cytokine effects	++	?+
Response to immunomodulation	+++	++ → +++

+, mild relationship; ++, moderate relationship; +++, strong relationship; ?, contradictory responses studies. Recent studies of an APL of the immunodominant portion of MBP revealed that in some MS patients, there was a suggestion of a shift to Th2, but also a tendency to cutaneous hypersensitivity responses.[8] More interestingly, in another group, three patients had up-regulation of an MBP reactive Th1 response, associated with exacerbations of MS and increased MRI activity.[9] These studies suggest that for APL to be a reasonable approach, it may need to be screened in individual patients to determine whether they will respond with a Th1 or Th2 response. Another important result of these studies is that they demonstrate an important role for MBP reactive cells in the immunopathogenesis of MS. One of the putative mechanisms of glatiramer acetate also invokes this mechanism of Th1 to Th2 switching. These therapeutic approaches have been demonstrated to produce an antigen-specific induction of Th2 cells which then migrate to the CNS where they "see" their cognate antigen, upregulate and secrete immunosuppressive cytokines which turn off any immune response in the proximity to the Th2 cells, even responses directed against other CNS antigens. This is referred to as "bystander suppression."[10]

However, while EAE is clearly an autoimmune response to an inciting agent, in MS the putative inciting antigen is unknown. Several components of myelin are suspect (MBP, PLP, myelin-oligodendrocyte glycoprotein), but none have been shown to unequivocally be the autoimmune target in MS, although the APL studies referenced above implicate MBP. Further, EAE is induced by inoculation with a myelin antigen, while MS appears to develop spontaneously, or at least without a clearly identifiable inciting cause.

The dysimmune state seen in MS provides further evidence for autoimmunity as the underlying pathogenic mechanism for MS (Table 2.3). Patients with MS have increased numbers of activated lymphocytes both in the peripheral circulation and in CSF. There is also evidence of decreased suppressor function. The presence of increased activation of immunocompetent cells and a decrease in the numbers of suppressor-inducer cells and functional suppressor activity would serve to produce a hyperimmune

Table 2.3 Immunologic abnormalities in patients with MS.

Peripheral blood:
Loss of nonspecific suppressor cell function
Decreased numbers of suppressor-inducer lymphocytes
Increased number of activated lymphocytes

Within the central nervous system:
Elevated levels of gamma globulin
Oligoclonal banding of IgG
Increased ratio of helper-inducer to suppressor-inducer lymphocytes
Increased number of activated lymphocytes
Different lymphocytic activation properties from blood

state, suitable for the development of an autoimmune disease. However, it is not yet known how these defects produce CNS autoreactivity. There are many studies reporting abnormalities of immune function, immune cellular components, and immunologic marker molecules, but none has proven to be consistent enough to define the immunologic abnormality of MS. Within the CNS, the most consistent, and diagnostically useful, abnormalities found are those of intra-CNS immunoglobulin production. This is manifest by elevated levels of immunoglobulin in cerebrospinal fluid (CSF) and an elevation in the ratio of immunoglobulin to other serum proteins in the CSF, indicating that the immunoglobulin is produced within the CNS. The immunoglobulin found within the CNS is usually oligoclonal in nature. This implies that a restricted number of plasma cell clones are producing anti-body within the CNS. In several other diseases demonstrating CSF oligo-clonal bands, such as subacute sclerosing panencepalitis (SSPE), the antigen that the oligoclonal antibody is directed against is known. In MS, the antigen that the oligoclonal bands might react with is unknown, despite extensive studies. An oligoclonal banding pattern is also found in the immunoglobulin eluted from brain tissue of patients with MS.

The immunopathological cascade (Figure 2.7) that may lead to MS involves the sensitization of CD4+T cells in the periphery, via presentation

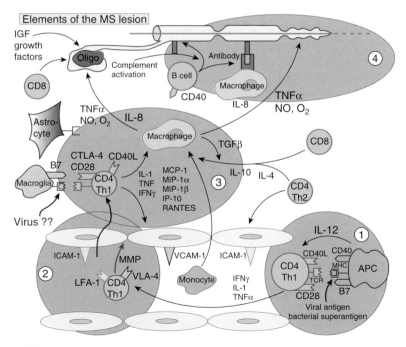

Figure 2.7
A simplified model of the immunological cascade in multiple sclerosis. Numbered zones represent potential therapeutic targets. (courtesy of Dr H. McFarland).

of an autoantigen by an antigen presenting cell to specific T cell receptor bearing lymphocytes which then traffic to the CNS (activated T cells readily pass through the blood–brain barrier but likely interact with adhesion molecules on the cerebrovascular endothelium) and upregulate in response to "seeing" their cognate antigen, presented by a CNS antigen presenting cell, likely a macrophage or microglial cell (although astrocytes and CNS endothelial cells potentially may present antigen). On upregulating, these CD4+Th1 cells secrete IFN-γ, IL-2, TNF, other cytokines and chemokines (small molecular chemoattractants), cause breakdown of the blood–brain barrier with attendant increase in cellular trafficking and activate microglia which then can directly damage myelin and oligodendrocytes or lead to the production of molecules that mediate tissue damage, e.g., nitric oxide, free radicals, or possibly complement. The immune response would be downregulated by Th2 cells, secreting IL-4, IL-10, and transforming growth factor (TGF). The damage could be part of a directed autoimmune response or secondary to nonspecific damage to myelin/ oligodendrocytes by the products of the immune response — a bystander reaction[11] (Table 2.4).

The viral hypothesis arises from several lines of evidence. Epidemiological data suggests that MS may be an illness related to childhood exposure to an unknown agent that then expresses itself later in life. There are similarities between MS and virologic models of demyelination such as Theiler's murine encephalomyelitis virus infection (TMEV). TMEV infection in mice is followed by an immune-mediated chronic demyelinating condition that can be treated with immunosuppressant agents. Many microbes have been implicated in the pathogenesis of MS over the past several decades (spirochetes, measles virus, paramyxoviruses, HTLV-1, and others), but none has stood up to critical analysis. HTLV-1 infection of the CNS is intriguing in that it produces a chronic demyelinating condition, primarily of the spinal cord, that has similarities to MS, although there are clear differentiating features. More recently, interest has centered on the

Table 2.4 Immunologic pros and cons.

Pros:
MS dysimmune state
Successful Interferon studies
Glatiramer acetate
EAE
Pathology

Cons:
Anti-CD4–lack of therapeutic benefit
Anti-TNF–lack of therapeutic benefit, ? worsening of MS
Lack of convincing effect of most immunosuppressant therapy
Failure of oral myelin trial

virus HHV-6, although the association of this virus with MS is not yet compelling. Another agent under current investigation is *Chlamydia pneumoniae*, a bacterium, which has been isolated from the CNS of some MS patients.[12] This agent has also been associated with other pathogenic states, unrelated to MS. Thus its connection with MS remains unproven, at this time. Additional studies are underway to try to confirm an MS causal relationship with either of these agents.

The likeliest role of viruses in MS pathogenesis relates to the concept of molecular mimicry. Here, the virus is simulating an autoantigen, generating a CNS directed autoimmune cascade, as described above.[13] There are many examples of microbial proteins or peptides that are immunologically cross-reactive with portions of human organs. In the case of the CNS, a microbe could have cross-reacting sequences with immunodominant portions of a myelin antigen, such as myelin basic protein, proteolipid protein, myelin-oligodendrocyte glycoprotein, etc. The mechanism by which exposure to such an agent or agents leads to a state of CNS autoimmunity in some individuals and not others is not clear, but may relate, in part, to the immunogenetic makeup of the individual. Another potential mechanism of disease is by direct attack on oligodendroglia or myelin by a microorganism (Table 2.5).

Table 2.5 Potential immunopathogenic mechanisms of disease in MS.

Cell-mediated attack against CNS antigen
Bystander effects of nonspecific inflammation on myelin
Molecular mimicry by a microorganism
Viral attack on oligodendrocytes or myelin

Pathophysiology

The production of clinical symptoms and signs in MS results from alteration of the conductive properties of nerve fibers in the CNS. This may result from demyelination and/or axonal damage. The determination of whether an area of inflammatory demyelination is expressed clinically depends on where in the CNS the lesion occurs, i.e., the more eloquent the area, the more likely a lesion in that location will produce signs or symptoms. Equally important is whether the lesion alters the conductive properties of the damaged nerve fibers sufficiently to impede or block conduction. This will depend on whether the lesion is purely demyelinating or if axonal damage has occurred. In the latter case, conduction will fail. In the former, conduction may be slowed, with or without functional significance, depending on the degree of slowing and the safety factor of conduction.

Myelin serves as an insulator of the axon such that action potentials are not propagated along the length of the axon, but instead conduction

Conduction defect in demyelination

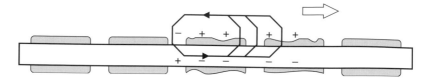

Figure 2.8

Saltatory conduction, ion channels. Loss of myelin impedes the effciency of saltatory conduction.

occurs from one node of Ranvier to the next. The concept of conduction jumping from one node to the next was first proposed by Lillie who coined the term "saltatory conduction" (Figure 2.8). This limitation of current flow to the nodal area allows for much faster conduction of neural impulses. In addition to speeding conduction, the presence of a myelin sheath allows for many fibers with high conduction velocity to be contained in a small area, e.g., a nerve trunk. Also myelin allows for energy conservation by limiting ionic flow to the nodal regions and also permits more rapid repetitive firing.

The conveyance of information by a single nerve fiber is accomplished primarily by the number of impulses propagated per unit time. The size of an action potential, i.e., its amplitude, is relatively constant. The impulse is either of sufficient amplitude to propagate the action potential along the axon or it is not; the all-or-none rule. Therefore, for any given nerve fiber the quantitative expression of signal intensity must be expressed by the frequency with which the nerve fires. As myelin plays an integral role in the conduction velocity of a nerve fiber, one can easily see how an alteration of the myelin sheath, and thus the speed of conduction, could have profound effects on signaling within the nervous system.

The distribution of axonal membrane ion channels in myelinated nerves differs from that of unmyelinated nerves. In unmyelinated nerves, there is a relatively uniform membrane distribution of voltage sensitive ion channels. Myelinated nerves, by contrast, demonstrate a more complex arrangement of ion channels. There is a high density of sodium channels at the nodes of Ranvier and a very low density of sodium channels along the internodal membrane (Figure 2.9). This corresponds with studies demonstrating that sodium currents are limited to the nodal membrane. Activation of sodium channels is necessary for propagation of action potentials, and their localization at the nodes of Ranvier is needed for saltatory conduction to occur. Potassium channels demonstrate a complementary localization along the axonal membrane, occurring at higher density along the internodal mem-

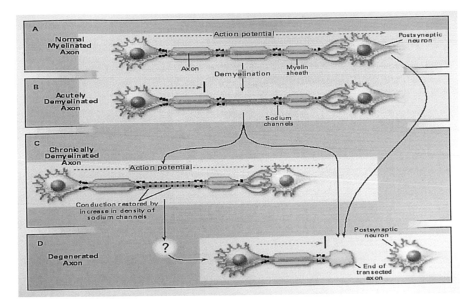

Figure 2.9
Acute and chronic molecular alteration in MS[14] (from Waxman, NEJM).

brane than at the nodes. In saltatory conduction, anything that increases current loss within the internode would be expected to delay activation of successive nodes of Ranvier, thereby prolonging internodal conduction time and reducing conduction velocity. Conduction through demyelinated internodes may be slowed by a factor of greater than 25.[15]

Conduction velocity will fail when the loss of current within the internode exceeds the safety factor of the nodal current of the intact nodes. The alteration of function seen as a result of delay in conduction can be understood best by recalling that signaling in the nervous system is critically dependent on maintenance of proper conduction velocity. It is possible that below a certain frequency a train of impulses no longer conveys utilizable information. Slowing of conduction can cause temporal dispersion of a signal, which may cause a loss of synchrony at the synapse distal to the deranged signal or may cause the loss of sufficient excitatory postsynaptic potentials to propagate an action potential at the next synapse. The net effect of this decrease in conduction velocity will vary depending on where in the nervous system the lesions are. Slowing of conduction can be seen in evoked potential studies in the absence of symptoms or signs. This is a possible explanation for the "silent" lesions seen in patients with MS.

Intermittent conduction block may occur due to the inability to conduct rapid trains of stimuli. Somatosensory evoked potential studies in MS patients have demonstrated this phenomenon. This conduction defect is likely to affect functions that depend on maintenance of precisely timed, prolonged bursts of impulses. This phenomenon may explain abnormalities in appreciation of vibration sense, fatigue during sustained motor activity, and certain intermittent visual abnormalities in patients with MS. In damaged nerve fibers, there is an increased sensitivity to changes in temperature and ionic milieu, such that conduction block will occur more readily than in normal fibers. This would explain the temperature sensitivity of many MS patients and Uhthoff's phenomenon (alteration in visual acuity during periods of exercise, likely due to increase in core body temperature).

Nerve conduction may also be adversely affected by circulating factors. These might explain the rapid production of symptoms and the equally rapid recovery that sometimes occurs, much more rapid than explained by remyelination. These factors are not well identified, but perhaps cytokines, edema, or antibodies might play a role.

Somewhat slower restoration of conduction, but still more rapid than explained by remyelination, occurs via diffuse upregulation of sodium channels on recently demyelinated axonal membrane, allowing restoration of conduction (Figure 2.9).

Remyelination occurs in some lesions as a result of regeneration of oligodendrocytes, arising either from remaining mature oligodendrocytes or from a precursor pool within the CNS. Schwann cells may also participate in remyelinating demyelinated regions close to peripheral nerve root entry zones in the spinal cord and brainstem. Remyelinated regions have thinner myelin sheaths (shadow plaques) and usually shorter internodal segments. Remyelination is typically incomplete and ultimately fails to keep up with the destructive process, leading to advancing disability.[16]

Paroxysmal and positive phenomena may result from several mechanisms of hyperexcitability: spontaneous ectopic excitation; mechanically evoked excitation; autoexcitation arising from previous activity in the same nerve; and ephaptic excitation (cross-talk). The occurrence of spontaneous and mechanically induced discharges has been proposed as the mechanism for the development of some of the paroxysmal and "positive" symptoms seen in patients with MS. The spontaneous activity was felt to provide an explanation for the prolonged paresthesias and the facial myokymia. Small deformations of less than 1 mm at the site of spinal lesions could increase spontaneous activity and transiently induced ectopic activity in quiescent fibers. This mechanically evoked activity would appear to be a good explanation for the occurrence of paresthesias radiating down the spine and into the legs and arms on flexing the neck that occurs in patients with cervical spinal cord disease (Lhermitte's phenomenon). On flexion and extension of the neck, the cervical spine changes its length by several centimeters, and therefore can supply sufficient stimulus for mechanically evoked activity. Ephaptic activity has been hypothesized as the cause for certain paroxysmal features seen in patients with MS, including tonic seizures, paroxysmal dysarthria and ataxia, and certain paroxysmal sensory abnormalities.

References

1. Trapp BD, Peterson J, Ransohoff RM, Rudick R, Mork S, Bo L. Axonal transection in the lesions of multiple sclerosis. N Engl J Med 1998; 338:278–285.

2. Ferguson B, Matyszak MK, Esiri MM, Perry VH. Axonal damage in acute multiple sclerosis lesions. Brain 1997; 120(Pt 3):393–399.

3. Lucchinetti C, Bruck W, Parisi J, Scheithauer B, Rodriguez M, Lassmann H. Heterogeneity of multiple sclerosis lesions: implications for the pathogenesis of demyelination. Ann Neurol 2000; 47:707–717.

4. Kalman B, Lublin FD. Immunopathogenic mechanisms in experimental allergic encephalomyelitis. Curr Opin Neurol Neurosurg 1993; 6:182–188.

5. Martin R. Immunological aspects of experimental allergic encephalomyelitis and multiple sclerosis and their application for new therapeutic strategies. J Neural Transmission 1997; 49(suppl):53–67.

6. Genain CP, Nguyen MH, Letvin NL, et al. Antibody facilitation of multiple sclerosis-like lesions in a nonhuman primate. J Clin Invest 1995; 96:2966–2974.

7. Martino G, Hartung HP. Immunopathogenesis of multiple sclerosis: the role of T cells. Curr Opin Neurol 1999; 12:309–321.

8. Kappos L, Comi G, Panitch H, et al. Induction of a non-encephalitogenic type 2 T helper-cell autoimmune response in multiple sclerosis after administration of an altered peptide ligand in a placebo-controlled, randomized phase II trial. Nat Med 2000; 6:1176–1182.

9. Bielekova B, Goodwin B, Richert N, et al. Encephalitogenic potential of the myelin basic protein peptide (amino acids 83–99) in multiple sclerosis: results of a phase II clinical trial with an altered peptide ligand. Nat Med 2000; 6:1167–1175.

10. Neuhaus O, Farina C, Yassouridis A, et al. Multiple sclerosis: comparison of copolymer-1-reactive T cell lines from treated and untreated subjects reveals cytokine shift from T helper 1 to T helper 2 cells. Proc Natl Acad Sci USA 2000; 97:7452–7457.

11. Hohlfeld R. Immunological basis for the therapy of multiple sclerosis. Acta Neurol Belg 1999; 99:40–43.

12. Sriram S, Mitchell W, Stratton C. Multiple sclerosis associated with Chlamydia pneumoniae infection of the CNS. Neurology 1998; 50:571–572.

13. Grogan JL, Kramer A, Nogai A, et al. Cross-reactivity of myelin basic protein-specific T cells with multiple microbial peptides: experimental autoimmune encephalomyelitis induction in TCR transgenic mice. J Immunol 1999; 163:3764–3770.

14. Waxman SG. Demyelinating diseases – new pathological insights, new therapeutic targets. N Engl J Med 1998; 338:323–325.

15. Moll C, Mourre C, Lazdunski M, Ulrich J. Increase of sodium channels in demyelinated lesions of multiple sclerosis. Brain Res 1991; 556:311–316.

16. Lassmann H, Bruck W, Lucchinetti C, Rodriguez M. Remyelination in multiple sclerosis. Mult Scler 1997; 3:133–136.

3
Epidemiology and genetics

For well over a century, since the early clinical and pathological descriptions of multiple sclerosis, investigators have struggled to determine the etiology of this seemingly capricious and, at times, devastating illness. To date, this search has brought many hints, but no definitive answers. For several decades now a variety of epidemiological studies have been conducted in order to provide clues to causation. In more recent years, attention has also been focused on the importance of genetic factors in the disease. A plethora of studies in both these areas has provided abundant data, not always consistent, yielding tantalizing possibilities, but ultimately, as yet, no resolution of the mystery.

Descriptive epidemiological studies in MS are plagued by some key diagnostic issues.[1-3] First of all, any successful investigation of the occurrence of a disease requires accuracy of diagnosis. MS remains a clinical diagnosis, with no simple laboratory investigation available that reliably certifies a case. At times definitive diagnosis is elusive or misdiagnosis may occur, leading to erroneous data. The likelihood is greater that cases are underrecognized than overrecognized in most surveys. The availability and refinement of MRI techniques are already helping to improve the reliability of case ascertainment. Furthermore, epidemiological studies, in general, are subject to the risk of biased case ascertainment. For example, is the record-keeping or diagnostic acumen equivalent in one area to another?

Incidence and prevalence

Many investigators have examined the occurrence of MS in a variety of geographic locations. The incidence of a disease refers to the number of new cases of that entity occurring per unit of time (in the case of MS usually 1 year) and population (with MS, usually 100,000). By contrast, "prevalence" refers to the number of cases present (alive) at any particular time (referred to as "prevalence day") within a defined population. The ratio of cases to population is termed the point prevalence rate or prevalence ratio.[1-4]

In general, it is significantly more difficult to obtain accurate incidence information than prevalence data. This is particularly true for MS because of frequent uncertainty about the date of onset, the lag time between first symptoms and actual diagnosis, and the uncertainty of diagnosis in early stages of the disease. As a result of these problems, most MS epidemiological studies have either been limited to prevalence data or have made inferences about incidence rates from a combination of prevalence and mortality data.

Prevalence is easier to determine than incidence because all cases are included regardless of duration. Nonetheless, the issues cited above may remain important. An additional consideration is the fact that major changes in birth rates can influence the crude prevalence rates, particularly for a disease like MS which is not evenly distributed across the life span. Thus, it is important that studies determine age-specific prevalence rates whenever possible.

Over the years many studies have determined the prevalence of MS in a variety of locales throughout the world. While many more studies, with generally more reliable data, have been conducted in the Northern Hemisphere, data are available as well from the Southern Hemisphere. Kurtzke has examined many of these surveys and classified rates as high (>30/100,000 – usually between 50 and 120), medium (5–29/100,000), and low (<5/100,000).[4,5] Included among the high prevalence areas are much of northern and central Europe (Figure 3.1), Italy, the northern United States, Canada, southeastern Australia, parts of the former Soviet Union, and New Zealand. Within the medium range are southern Europe, the southern United States, northern Australia, northernmost Scandinavia, much of the northern Mediterranean basin, parts of the former Soviet Union, white South Africa, and possibly central South America. Categorized in the low prevalence group are areas, where data are known, in Africa, Asia, and the Caribbean, Mexico and possibly northern South America

As a general rule, there is a diminishing north to south gradient for MS prevalence in the northern hemisphere [4,5] Conversely, in the southern hemisphere an increasing prevalence rate exists from north to south. For example, the prevalence of MS in the United States increases approximately two- to threefold as one examines data, for example, from southern states to the northern tier. Kurtzke's figures, however, suggest a range of prevalence from 90/100,000 in the northwestern states to 17/100,000 in the southeastern states (Figure 3.2). Another way to view the geographic prevalence differences is to consider that, in general, MS is more prevalent in temperate climates among more economically developed countries of the west.

Much of the latitude effect, especially in the northern hemisphere, may result from ethnic variation in susceptibility (see below). In both Europe and the United States, prevalence tends to reflect the degree of

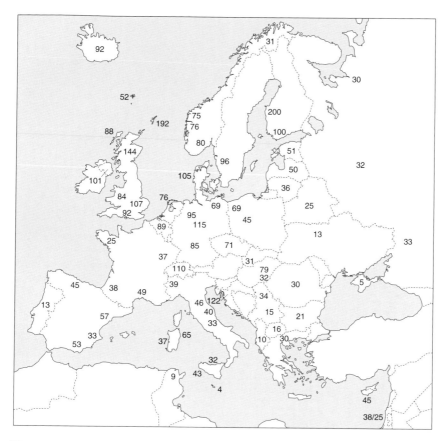

Figure 3.1
Prevalence of multiple sclerosis in Europe. (Redrawn from Kurtzke, 2001).[4]

Scandinavian and northern European heritage within the resident population.[6,7] Poser, in an extensive historic treatise, has suggested that modern distribution of MS may be the result of Viking raids in the middle ages leading to the introduction of susceptibility genes into native populations.[8]

However, exceptions occur to this possible explanation. For example, although no significant ethnic gradient has been identified in Australia, a fourfold difference nonetheless exists between the relatively low prevalence area of Queensland in the north and the higher prevalence area of Hobart, Tasmania in the south (Figure 3.3). [9,10] Ethnically similar populations live in London, Ontario where the prevalence rate is 94 and in Queensland, Australia where it is only 18.[11] Interestingly, even in Japan where the overall prevalence is low, the north–south gradient exists.

Thus, the implications of geographic prevalence data are far from simple and are complicated by a number of additional observations. One additional consideration is the fact that even within a given geographic

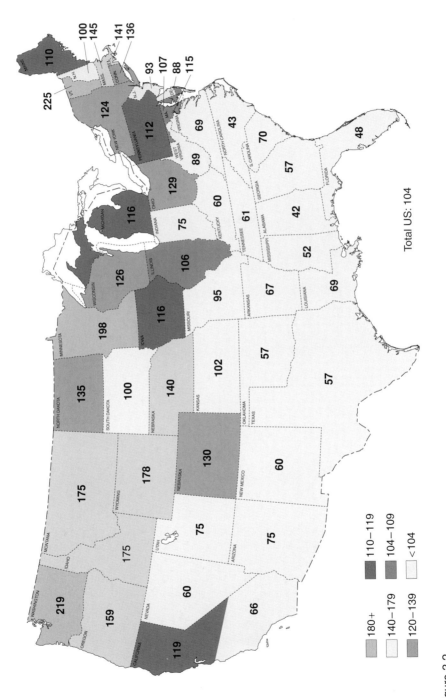

Figure 3.2
Prevalence of multiple sclerosis in the United States (Redrawn from Kurtzke, 2001).[4]

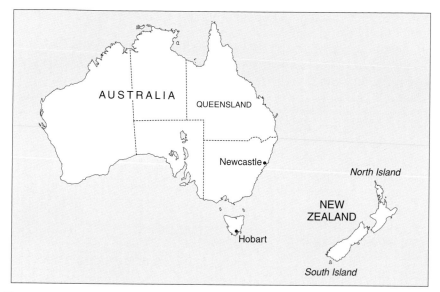

Figure 3.3
Map of Australia. A fourfold difference in prevalence exists between the northern area of Queensland and the southern area of Hobart, Tasmaina.

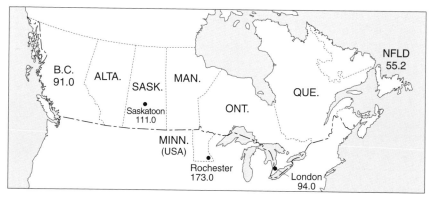

Figure 3.4
Prevalence of multiple sclerosis in areas of Canada and the northern United States demonstrating variation in rates even in locations with comparable latitude and climate (Redrawn from Ebers and Sadounick, 1998).[1]

area of comparable latitude and climate – for example the northern United States and Canada – prevalence rates may vary substantially. Thus the rates are 173 in Rochester, Minnesota; 111 in Saskatchewan; 94 in London, Ontario; 91 in British Columbia; and only 55 in Newfoundland (Figure 3.4).[1] An even more striking example of variation within a general geographic region is the comparison between a prevalence of 4.2 on the island of Malta and a rate of 53.3 found by the same investigators only 3 years earlier in neighboring Sicily (Figure 3.5).[12,13] Other countries where substantial regional differences have been described include Norway, the United Kingdom, and Switzerland.

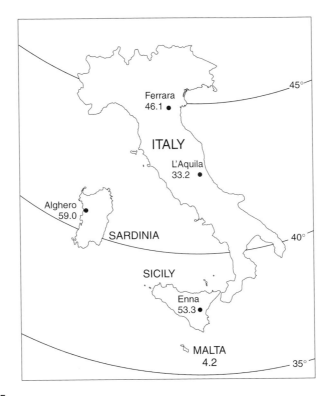

Figure 3.5
Prevalence in Malta is much lower than that in nearby Italian locations (Redrawn from Ebers and Sadounick, 1998).[1]

Correlational studies

A large number of correlational or ecological studies have been reported in MS.[3] This type of investigation can be particularly valuable in a disease such as MS because of its variable occurrence and especially when the variable of interest has relatively small differences within a small subpopulation. Weaknesses of the ecological approach are difficulties in documenting exact exposure, need to rely on proxy measures for exposure, and potential failure to identify an ethnic influence.

Among the factors correlating with MS prevalence is low temperature, demonstrated in numerous studies. Many investigations have also found a correlation between humidity and rainfall (particularly winter precipitation) and MS. The presence of coniferous forests and the content of peat in the soil have also been correlated. Industrialization, in general, but no particular industry, has been positively correlated with MS.

The influence of diet has frequently been examined, with studies correlating higher meat consumption and dairy food consumption with MS. Further, a correlation with processed and smoke-cured meat has been noted.

It must be emphasized that correlations by no means imply causation. The caveats mentioned above, particularly ethnic considerations, must be seriously regarded.

Race and ethnicity

Arguing against the primacy of environment as a critical factor determining the occurrence of MS are the striking differences in the prevalence among individuals of differing racial or ethnic backgrounds even living within the same geographic regions. Multiple sclerosis is very rare among African blacks, yet the disease occurs in African-Americans at a rate approximately half that of white Americans.[4] This difference most likely reflects the social admixture which takes place among the American population. Similarly, the disease is virtually unknown among native Americans (Amerindians), occurring exclusively among persons of mixed Amerindian and European heritage.

A number of other relatively isolated ethnic groups experience complete or nearly complete immunity from the disease. These include Eskimos, Yakutes, Hutterites, Norwegian Lapps, Hungarian Gypsies, Australian Aborigines, and New Zealand Maoris.[1,11]

Another interesting phenomenon apparently associated with race is an effect on the clinical expression of MS. This has been noted most strikingly in Japan, an area of generally low prevalence, where the disease far more commonly involves the optic nerves and spinal cord, rather than other areas of the central nervous system such as the brainstem, cerebellum, and cerebrum. This opticospinal form of MS, which occurs in other parts of Asia as well, is also frequently characterized by normal cranial MRI, a feature seldom found in European and North American cases of the disease.

Migrant studies

The observations of substantial differences in prevalence of MS among different geographic regions naturally led to interest in exploring the effects of migration on the occurrence of the disease. Numerous studies have been published reporting the results of investigations of migrants both from high risk areas to low risk areas and, conversely, from areas of low prevalence to those of high prevalence.

Conclusions, or even inferences, from migration studies must be tempered by the fact that such studies are subject to many potential sources of error and bias. Ideally, incidence and prevalence rates should be well established for the regions of both origin and destination. Unfortunately, the reliability of the data at both locales is sometimes questionable. Valid migrant studies must be based on two fundamental tenets: first, that migrants are truly representative of the country from which they come; and second, that in the new homeland the new migrants distribute themselves randomly. In reality, these assumptions are rarely entirely true. Many differences between migrants and the population at large of their country of origin undoubtedly serve as potential confounders of such studies. These include differences in demographics, ethnicity, religion, socioeconomic status, and health. Indeed, patients with MS may have disabilities or health requirements that preclude migration and some countries do not allow persons with medical disease to immigrate. Historically, as emphasized by Ebers and Sadovnick,[1,11] the greatest migrations have been triggered by religious persecution, wars or other upheavals; and migrants are commonly selected for economic, social, religious, health-related, and even personality and anthropologic characteristics.

Case ascertainment in the immigrant group may differ from that of the indigenous population. Furthermore, the proper denominator for the immigrant population in a specific area may be difficult to quantify. Different sizes of the populations in the two countries may be an additional complicating factor. In addition, the age of migration may have an affect on MS rates. Thus, situations in which the age of migration occurs after the critical period of putative exposure to an etiologic agent may result in false conclusions.

The potential hazard of ignoring these considerations may be illustrated by one particular study of Vietnamese migrants to France, where their risk of developing MS increased. However, all migrants had a French parent – a factor enabling migration – whereas those individuals remaining in Vietnam presumably for the most part did not. This obvious genetic difference was disregarded, as the population in the Vietnam war was used to establish the expected prevalence of Vietnamese migrants to France.

With these many caveats in mind, it seems, nonetheless, fair to conclude that, in general, migration appears to alter the risk of MS, with immigrants tending to adopt the rates of their new place of residence. The change in risk may not be immediate and may, at times, only be noted in children or descendants of the immigrant population. Studies by Dean initially suggested that rates of MS among immigrants from the United Kingdom and Europe to South Africa did not differ from those of South African born descendants, English-speaking whites and Afrikaaners.[14] Further analysis revealed that those immigrating before age 15 acquired the lower risk of MS of the population indigenous to South Africa, whereas those migrating later in life retained the higher risk of European natives.[15] Other studies have indicated that MS remains rare among African, Asian, and West Indian immigrants to the United Kingdom, but becomes much more common in their children. These data again suggest the causative importance of an environmental factor(s) in the occurrence of MS. Case control studies among the US armed forces showed a north–south gradient and, to a lesser extent, a west–east gradient. It was felt that high case ascertainment was likely because of financial benefits available for individuals with a diagnosis of MS. Data supported an increased risk of MS for migration from south to north and vice versa, but the risk appeared to change with older age of migration. However, at the time of these studies, it was not possible to control for genetic factors. More recent analysis suggests that at least some of the variation in geographic distribution may be explained by ethnic factors, as similar north–south and west–east gradients exist for specific subpopulations of northern European origin.

A series of interesting investigations has examined the effects of immigration to Israel. Initial reports by Alter suggested that the risk of MS for European Ashkenazi Jews was lowered for those moving before the age of 15, but not for those immigrating at older ages.[16] However this information was only available for those immigrating after 1940. On prevalence day in 1960, the maximum age of this immigrant group was only 34 and the mean age was much younger than that for the period of greatest risk for MS. In an attempt to address this problem, investigators subsequently examined age-specific prevalence in immigrants from Africa and Asia (Sephardic Jews) and then found that Europeans who immigrated after the age of 15 had much higher prevalence rates than the Sephardim, whereas those who immigrated at younger ages did not. The situation is further complicated by a recent reevaluation which indicated that Israeli born children of immigrants from Europe and America have MS rates comparable to those of their parents. These data suggest that genetic factors play a more important role than environmental determinants in this population. However, further observations that Israeli born children of Sephardic Jews have a higher prevalence of MS than would be expected from the prevalence rates of their parents' lands of origin again suggests an important environmental influence. These apparently conflicting observations only serve to underscore the extreme complexity involved in analyzing the dynamic between genetic and environmental influences. Each seems to play a role in determining the development of MS. The Israeli data further emphasize the difficulties inherent in conducting valid epidemiological studies in this disease and making accurate inferences from them.

Other migrant studies also seem to confirm the interplay between genetic and environmental determinants. Thus, Japanese and other Asians retain a relatively low risk of MS after immigrating to the United States. Nevertheless, the rate of MS among US Japanese is higher than that for those remaining in Japan.[17] Furthermore, Japanese born in Hawaii retain a low risk of MS and a predominance of opticospinal forms of the disease. By contrast, Hawaiian born Caucasians experience a lower rate of MS than those born elsewhere. Native Hawaiians do not develop MS, whereas mixed Hawaiian-Caucasians do.[18]

In summary, the results of migration studies yield an unclear message, but one offering some support for a role of both genetic and environmental factors. There is certainly, at least from a number of studies, evidence to suggest that an environmental exposure early in life in genetically susceptible persons may cause MS. However, susceptible individuals in low risk areas do seem to retain vulnerability. Looking at the data collectively, several investigators have postulated the "polio hypothesis." By analogy to the situation clearly established for polio, they have suggested that the putative environmental factor, whatever it may be, is ubiquitous in low prevalence areas. In these regions, early exposure to the agent is disease protective whereas delayed exposure in areas where the agent is less frequently encountered results in higher risk of clinical disease. While this hypothesis remains provocative, no direct evidence exists in its support.

Clusters

Clusters, defined as an excess of disease occurrence in a particular geographic area, have served as another argument in favor of an environmental determinant of MS. A number of such clusters have been described in MS, including occurrences in Key West, Florida; Henribourg, Saskatchewan; Colchester County, Nova Scotia; Vaasa, Finland; Hordaland, Norway; Los Alamos, New Mexico; Mansfield, Massachusetts; and among workers in a zinc-related manufacturing plant.[3,5] Probably the world's highest prevalence rates occur in the Orkney and Shetland Islands off Scotland. In the former, but not the latter, additional clustering occurs in time and space. Data showed clustering occurring 21 or more years before onset and, alternatively, just before onset of MS. Each of these two time clusters appeared in three separate islands.

The analysis of clusters, like that of migration studies, is troubled by several problems. These include: ascertainment biases; so-called bandwagon effects; misdiagnosis; the possibility that large kindreds of MS in a small community may be the cause; and determination that suspected exposure actually occurred before disease onset. The most critical issue casting doubt on the utility of cluster studies is statistical:

> Armon et al have reviewed how one might discriminate between bonafide cluster and chance by rigorous exclusion of the null hypothesis; this approach is based on correction of the P value for the number of implicit comparisons that are made. For example, if one observes an excess number of cases in a given county in the United States, one must adjust the P value for the number of estimated com-

parisons in other counties of the United States, where, presumably, a similar excess has not been found.[3]

When all these factors are considered, one must conclude that little useful information can be derived from the cluster reports currently available.

Epidemics

In contrast to clusters in a particular geographic area, disease clusters in time argue strongly for a transmissible environmental agent. By far the most studied apparent epidemic has been that described by Kurtzke et al in the Faroe Islands. These islands, formerly a Danish possession, are situated between Iceland and Norway.[19-22] The inhabitants receive their medical care in Denmark, enabling thorough acquisition of their medical records. In the original reports, the authors reported no cases of MS occurring prior to World War II. By contrast, they reported 46 cases occurring between 1943 and 1982, with an additional four cases between 1986 and 1989 (Figure 3.6). These data yielded point prevalence rates of 41 in 1950, 64 in 1961, 38 in 1972, and 34 in 1977. The investigators interpreted the data to suggest a point source epidemic related to the stationing of 8000 British troops in the Faroe Islands, beginning in 1941. Their further work suggested that this military deployment actually triggered four consecutive, albeit declining, epidemics, the fourth consisting of seven patients with symptom onset between 1984 and 1989. Analyses of birth cohorts revealed that the initial epidemic involved postpubescent individuals greater than 11 years of age in 1941 and that subsequent epidemics involved those who had been younger than 11.

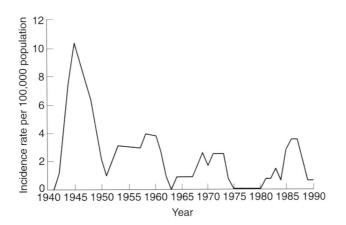

Figure 3.6
Four epidemics of MS in the Faroe Islands, where MS had not been reported prior to the occupation by British troops in the 1940's. (From Kurtzke, 2001).[4]

Despite the intensive analysis and description of the Faroe Islands "epidemic" by Kurtzke and coworkers, several authors have argued strongly against its validity. The critics have suggested that MS may have existed before the British occupation and that its apparent rarity may have been the result of poor case ascertainment which improved after World War II. Furthermore, a retrospective study commencing 30 years after the fact is problematic and dating the clinical onset of MS under such circumstances may be particularly difficult. In addition, because of the small number of cases, misdating the clinical onset of a single case would significantly affect the incidence rate. The original reports also lack good case-control data with respect to the degree of exposure to British troops.

A second, but less convincing epidemic in Iceland, also in relation to the presence of British troops during World War II, was described.[23] The average annual incidence between 1945 and 1954 was 3.2/100,000, compared with 1.6 between 1923 and 1944, and 1.9 between 1955 and 1974. The situation differed from the Faroes because MS did exist before the British occupation. An important potential confounding factor is that one of the authors of the report was the first neurologist in Iceland, arriving in 1942, which may have influenced the apparent increase of MS over the next few years. This may have been particularly true for earlier detection of mild cases in young Icelanders.

These important critiques notwithstanding, the reports of the apparent Faroese epidemic stand as provocative arguments in favor of an environmental determinant of MS. In particular, they bolster the belief of many that a particular virus may be the etiologic agent for MS. Even if the epidemic is valid and a critical infectious agent was introduced into a susceptible population, the implication that the same factor is operative elsewhere, in other cases of MS, may not be justified. Furthermore, an alternative possibility, as suggested by Ebers and Sadovnick, is that the introduction of a large number of common viruses into a virgin susceptible population might trigger an apparent epidemic without the implication of a specific transmissible agent.[1]

Temporal patterns

A number of geographic regions have been surveyed for prevalence or incidence on more than one occasion. Most of these studies have showed an apparent increase in these figures, although exceptions demonstrating a decrease have also been reported.

Before considering the details of these investigations, however, it is important once again to indicate the potential pitfalls. Prevalence changes over time may be influenced by one or more of the following factors:

1. different methodologies
2. changing definitions of MS
3. different investigators
4. different awareness of MS
5. earlier recognition of cases
6. changing diagnostic accuracy
7. prolonged survival
8. differences in population structure
9. migration of patients into or inability to emigrate from an area.

Increased incidence rates may be the result of improved diagnostic capabilities, genetic susceptibility, environmental factors, or migration from a high prevalence area.

The most reliable data on changes in incidence come prospectively when an institution provides ongoing care to a population base and where access to health care is not limited by socioeconomic factors. Such is the case in Olmsted County, Minnesota, where the incidence has increased over each of the last three decades to a rate of 7–8/100,000. In Sassari, Sardinia, where incidence has been tracked in triennia since 1965, the incidence increased from 2/100,000 in 1965–1977 to over 5 after 1977.[1,24] In Hordaland county in western Norway, the incidence for clinically definite and probable MS appears to have increased from 1.12 in 1953–1957 to 3.5 in 1973.[25] Elsewhere in Norway, in More and Romsdad counties, the incidence doubled from 1.94 in 1950–1954 to 3.78 in 1975–1979.[26]

Studies also showed an increasing prevalence rate in Saskatoon, Canada. Ebers and Sadovnick, however, commented that "improved survival, the availability of various diagnostic tests to assist in the diagnosis of MS, and the institution of the universal coverage medical insurance program in Canada all contributed to the apparent rise in prevalence."[1] Subsequent studies also showed comparable prevalence rates throughout Canada with the exception of Newfoundland

Declining incidence, however, has been noted in some areas. The incidence rate in Gothenburg, Sweden was stable at 4.2/100,000 between 1950 and 1964, but fell to 2.7 and 2.0, respectively, in two 5-year periods ending in 1988. A decline in incidence was noted in the very high prevalence area of the Orkney Islands between 1951 and 1968. Although most prevalence studies have shown an increase in a second survey, exceptions have occurred in Manitoba (Winnipeg), Canada, and in western Poland.

Sex ratio

Although some variation occurs among different surveys, the female:male ratio tends to approach 2:1 in population studies. This ratio appears to be further increased in early onset cases, although postmenopausal onset does not seem to change the sex ratio. The female preponderance is possibly further increased in familial cases and in individuals positive for HLA-DR2.

Age of onset

The most widely applied diagnostic criteria of Poser et al[27] employed an age of onset range of 10–59, compared to earlier studies which used an upper age limit of 50. However, cases are clearly described both in childhood and older age. Duquette found that 2.7% of cases at his center occurred before the age of 16 and these younger cases had a higher female : male ratio of 3 : 1.[28] Perhaps more than 5% of cases occur in older individuals even into the eighth decade.

Recent studies have shown a correlation between age of onset in sibling pairs concordant for MS. Furthermore, stronger correlation was seen for concordant monozygotic twin pairs than for nontwin MS sibling pairs, indicating that age of onset in MS may be partly under genetic control.

Quest for an infectious agent

Some of the epidemiological investigations cited above have naturally fueled interest in the possibility that MS is caused by an infectious agent. Most attention has focused on a potential viral etiology[29] and a current hypothesis melds this possibility with the autoimmune nature of the disease. This viewpoint suggests that a virus initiates the autoimmune process through the phenomenon of "molecular mimicry", in which a viral antigen shares a recognition site with a component of a myelin protein so that the immune defense against the former also results in damage to myelin. Numerous viruses have been nominated over the years as the causative agent for MS, as listed in Table 3.1, but none has been validated in subsequent investigations.

When analyzing claims of responsibility for a particular infectious agent, one must be attentive to a variety of possible landmines. Did the investigators include adequate control subjects, including those with other neurological disease? Were the control materials collected in the same fashion as the MS materials? Was the investigator blinded and were the samples coded? Were the investigators sensitive to the possibility of laboratory contamination and were the pitfalls of new technology recognized? This has become particularly true with the availability of polymerase chain reaction technology, a highly sensitive analytical tool, but one easily subject to laboratory contamination.

Table 3.1 Viruses that could be causative agents for MS.

Virus
• Rabies
• Herpes simplex virus
• Scrapie
• Measles
• Parainfluenza
• "Carp agent"
• "MS agent"
• Paramyxovirus
• Simian cytomegalovirus
• Corona virus
• Canine distemper virus
• HTLV-1
• Human herpesvirus 6
• Epstein–Barr virus

Although not substantiated, over the years a number of provocative suggestions relating to viral agents have been made. After reports by Cook and colleagues of a positive correlation between dog ownership, suggesting an association with canine distemper virus,[30,31] a host of case-control studies were undertaken to examine a possible relationship to animal exposure. While the majority of these studies have been negative, some have shown more exposure among MS patients to dogs (in general), indoor dogs, small dogs, or dog exposure in the 5–10 year period prior to MS diagnosis. Cook has argued that these studies are insensitive because of a high baseline rate of exposure to dogs. Higher antibody titers to measles virus, another myxovirus, in MS patients raised the possibility of a causal relationship. However, no convincing differences have been found when appropriate control studies have been done. The previously discussed declining incidence of MS in Gothenburg, Sweden was considered possibly related to measles eradication. Nevertheless, recent studies have demonstrated that the majority of young MS patients have been immunized to measles virus and thus have antibodies raised agains this live virus vaccine.

Members of the herpes virus group have also received considerable attention as potential causes of MS or, at least, specific triggers of exacerbations. One proposal raised the possibility that the extreme rarity of MS among Canadian Hutterites was secondary to a relatively low rate for infections by herpes zoster.[6,32] Recent reports of a role for human herpesvirus 6, an extremely common and usually asymptomatic infection of childhood which does cause exanthem subitum, have been widely publicized.[33] At least one report has failed to demonstrate a statistically significant decrease in MS exacerbation rate after treatment with acyclovir.

HTLV-1 infection has generated interest because of its association with a myelopathic disorder (HTLV-1 associated myelopathy, sometimes known as tropical spastic paraparesis). Whereas this syndrome may resemble MS, it differs clinically and in its neuroimaging manifestations from usual MS cases, who do not otherwise manifest evidence of HTLV-1 infection.

Recent attention has centered on a possible association of MS with *Chlamydia pneumoniae*, a bacterial agent causing at times a generally mild pneumonia. Using PCR techniques, the agent was reported to be present much more frequently in MS patients than in controls.[34-36] However, once again confirmation of these findings has not yet been forthcoming.

At the present time, it seems likely that most reports of increased antibody titers to various agents in MS reflect heightened immunoreactivity in this disease population. Furthermore, viral infections, in general, probably serve to trigger MS exacerbations, rather than to cause the disease. Minor respiratory infections preceded relapse in 27% of patients, the only significant factor identified in association with exacerbation, in one cohort study. Other studies have reported a seasonal increase in relapses during the months when respiratory infections are more common. In the successful pivotal trial of glatiramer acetate for the treatment of relapsing-remitting MS, viral infection was again identified as an apparent precipitant of attacks.[37] The mechanism by which viral infection may stimulate relapse may be through release of interferon gamma, a cytokine which has been shown to be a potent precipitant of MS attacks.

Precipitating factors

Through the years a host of possible precipitating factors either for the onset of MS or new exacerbations have been suggested in addition to infection. These have included both emotional and physical stress, trauma, surgery and anesthesia, diet, heavy metals, overexertion or fatigue, and heat. None of these, however, has been validated by proper scientific investigation.

Most attention has been given to the possible roles of physical trauma or emotional stress. Difficulties are encountered in examining this issue because of the potential for "recall bias," the circumstance in which individuals with a particular condition, searching their memories for associations, may be more likely to recall such events as episodes of trauma. Several important studies, however, have failed to demonstrate an association between MS and physical trauma. Historic cohort studies can be conducted in centers that have a number of defined cohorts, especially a cohort of MS patients and a cohort with the defined putative risk factor. Such a situation exists at the Mayo Clinic, where analysis showed no relationship between head injury or lumbar disk surgery with the onset of MS, nor any demonstrable association between episodes of trauma and exacerbations,[38] findings consistent with earlier studies.[39] A recent thorough assessment of the available evidence led the Therapeutics and Technology Subcommittee of the American Academy of Neurology to conclude that there is no association between physical trauma and MS.[40]

The implications of emotional stress are more difficult to reconcile, in part because of the problems in rating the severity of stressful situations. While patients themselves very frequently believe that such stress has led to worsening of their neurological condition, little evidence currently supports that contention. Nonetheless, the possibility remains and the American Academy of Neurology report recently concluded that a possible relationship between emotional stress and MS has neither been established nor refuted at the present time.[40]

The effects of pregnancy on MS have been investigated in many studies. Most of these have been retrospective and suggested an increased relapse rate after parturition. Recently a large prospective study confirmed this impression, demonstrating a decline in exacerbation during pregnancy, but a statistically significant increase in relapse rate during the first three postpartum months.[41] This was in contrast to an earlier report which found no association either with pregnancy or the 6-month period after delivery and MS relapse.

Genetics

An unequivocally increased recurrence of MS in families could theoretically result from either genetic factors or a shared environmental situation. However, abundant evidence now exists to support the preeminence of genetic determinants as the explanation for this phenomenon.

The most persuasive data come from twin studies which show a markedly higher concordance rate in monozygotic twins than in dizygotic pairs. Ebers et al in a large twin study initially found a concordance rate among monozygotic twins of 26% compared to 2.4% in dizygotic twins.[42] When the cohort was further followed beyond the period of highest risk (age >50), the concordance rate rose to 30.8% for monozygotic twins compared to 4.7% for dizygotic twins. It has also been demonstrated that the apparently clinically unaffected twin often shows abnormal findings on MRI, evoked potential studies, or CSF examination, indicating the presence of subclinical disease. The high concordance rate in monozygotic twins does not necessarily imply a genetic influence. It should be noted that paralytic polio and tuberculosis, clearly caused by environmentally acquired pathogens, both have higher concordance rates in monozygotic than in dizygotic twins. Nonetheless, the difference does argue much more strongly for a major genetic determinant of MS.

The high monozygotic : dizygotic concordance ratio (approximately 10 : 1) supports a polygenic mode of inheritance. Were the disease determined by a simple autosomal dominant gene, a ratio of 2:1 would be expected. If a purely autosomal recessive pattern existed, the expected ratio would be 4:1. However, if a simple genetic explanation for MS is true, the concordance rate for monozygotic twins would be much higher, presumably approaching 100%.

Overall, approximately 20% of MS patients can identify another first degree family member with MS. Prospective studies have shown prevalence rates as high as 5% for daughters and decreasing as one becomes more removed from the proband (Table 3.2).[43]

This dilution with increasing genetic distance from the MS patient would be highly unlikely to occur with a simple Mendelian pattern of inheritance and suggests involvement of several ($n = 4$–5) genes.

A large Canadian study also showed risk dilution for half siblings as shown in Table 3.3.[44] This same study addressed the possibility of an environmental effect, examining the prevalence among half siblings who lived apart, compared to those who lived together. Any significant difference found between those raised apart (1.06%) and those raised together (0.67%) indicated that any environmental factor was not operative directly at the family level. Furthermore, among 238 MS patients who were adopted near birth, only one case of MS was found among 1201 nonbiological first degree relatives, a rate similar to the overall Canadian prevalence rate of 0.1%.

If early exposure to an infectious agent over a short time were to confer protection against later MS (the polio hypothesis), then later born children in a family should be at lower risk. However, a report of 164 cases of spo-

Table 3.2 Prevalence rates for MS in family members.

Relationship	Prevalence
Parents	3%
Sons	1%
Daughters	5%
Siblings	4%
Aunts/uncles	2%
Nieces/nephews	2%
First cousins	1%

Table 3.3 Risk dilution for half siblings of patients with MS.

Relationship	Prevalence
Full brother	1.72%
Maternal half brother	0.57%
Paternal half brother	0.49%
Full sister	3.87%
Maternal half sister	1.58%
Paternal half sister	1.25%

radic MS found that birth order position did not differ between patients and well matched spousal controls.[45] Studies also have failed to demonstrate any evidence to suggest transmissibility between spouses. Investigations of conjugal MS also indicate that the risk for children is higher when MS exists on both maternal and paternal sides.

Affected sibling pairs usually have an onset of symptoms at different points in time, but they tend to have their initial clinical manifestations at approximately the same age. An even stronger correlation between age of onset is found among monozygotic twin pairs. These findings also suggest a genetic rather than an environmental influence.

Although the data cited above clearly suggest the importance of genetic factors in the causation of MS, the specific susceptibility genes have proved elusive. The clearest associations have been with certain HLA antigens. Most consistently documented has been an overrepresentation of HLA-DR2 antigen in western Caucasians. However, various class I and classs II genes have been associated with MS, differing among different populations. Clearly though, possession of a certain HLA type is neither sufficient nor essential for the development of MS. Furthermore, the HLA effect is less prominent in MS than in other autoimmune diseases, such as juvenile onset diabetes mellitus.

Many other gene candidates have been suggested. Among those rejected are: the interleukins and their receptors; interferons α, β, and γ; the IgG constant region; α_1 antitrypsin; and mitochondrial genes. A potential linkage between tumor necrosis factor α and MS is weakened by the known linkage dysequilibrium of these gene complexes with DR2.

Currently, an extensive multinational effort is attempting to identify susceptibility genes in MS, with attention focused on the sharing of gene markers by MS-affected sibling pairs or by patients from families with several affected members. Thus far, more than 90% of the human genome has been excluded for major gene linkages to MS. Many weak linkages have been identified and four or more chromosomal regions appear to be consistently linked with MS. The findings of these studies appear to be consistent with the conclusions from epidemiological studies, suggesting that there are four or five involved genes, each with a minor effect, but none with an overwhelming effect.[6]

Other autoimmune disorders

Many other autoimmune disorders have been reported to occur in association with MS. These include thyroid disease, systemic lupus erythematosus, myasthenia gravis, diabetes mellitus, ankylosing spondylitis, inflammatory bowel disease, and scleroderma. Certain families appear to have a genetic predisposition to autoimmune diseases. The linkage of these disorders to MS, however, appears only to be well established for autoimmune thyroid disease for which a detailed survey in Olmsted

County, Minnesota showed a statistically significant association with MS. A similar relationship was identified in Ontario, Canada. Many autoimmune disorders share characteristics with MS. For example, juvenile onset diabetes mellitus, familial psoriasis, Crohn's disease, and asthma have distinct population frequencies and geographic gradients, share similar treatment approaches, and tend to be more common in women.

Uveitis seems to be particularly common in MS, occurring in up to 5% in some series. It has also been associated with various infections and other autoimmune diseases, including Behçet's disease, toxoplasmosis, ankylosing spondylitis, sarcoidosis, and syphilis. Thus, the uveal tract, although not myelinated, does frequently participate in the inflammatory process.

When considering the relative importance of genetic and environmental factors in determining the development of MS, interesting observations about animal models of autoimmune disease should be noted. All models of autoimmune disease in mice show an oligogenic or polygenic inheritance of susceptibility and some offer provocative epidemiological lessons. Particularly striking is the situation of the nonobese diabetic mouse. Despite genetic homogeneity, when colonies of inbred mice are distributed around the world, the penetrance of diabetes is remarkably variable. For example, mice reared in Auckland, New Zealand did not develop diabetes, whereas all those reared in Edmonton, Canada did. It appears that penetrance is strongly influenced by diet and cleanliness of the environment in early life and by viral contamination of breeding colonies. When exposed to a germ-free environment in early life, mice uniformly express glycosuric diabetes.[46]

Conclusions

Sifting through the plethora of data leads to the inescapable conclusion that determination of MS results from a complex interplay of environmental and genetic factors. Despite more contemporary reanalyses, which suggest that ethnic distribution may explain as much as 60% of the geographic variation in the United States and Europe, a clear north–south gradient exists seemingly independent of genetic or racial factors. However, the fact that major differences in prevalence exist in the absence of a difference in latitude bespeaks the probability of significant genetic factors. Examples of this are the strikingly greater prevalence of MS in Sicily compared to Malta and the existence of very low or absent MS prevalence among certain ethnic groups within an area of otherwise high prevalence (e.g. Lapps and Canadian Hutterites).

The high (approximately 30%) concordance rate among monozygotic twin pairs, compared to that of dizygotic twins, provides strong indication, if not absolute proof, of a major genetic influence. Conversely, the 70% discordance provides further support for the existence of nongenetic factors.

Other familial and ethnic studies additionally bolster the genetic argument. However, the evidence overwhelmingly refutes simple genetic explanations, instead supporting the view that at least several susceptibility genes must be operative, with the major culprits remaining unidentified.

A variety of tantalizing evidence has suggested the possibility of an infectious cause or trigger for MS. Despite this, no consistent data have emerged in support of any specific virus or other pathogen. It now appears more likely that infection in general, rather than a particular agent, may act as a nonspecific stimulus to the immune system resulting in initiation of an MS exacerbation.

Clearly the future will bring additional epidemiological and genetic studies. Those most likely to be fruitful will be examinations of populations in which control of genetic factors is optimal.

References

1. Ebers G, Sadovnick AD. Epidemiology. In: Paty DS, Ebers GC, eds. Multiple sclerosis. Philadelphia: FA Davis; 1998: 5–28.

2. Hogencamp W, Rodriguez M, Weinshenker B. The epidemiology of multiple sclerosis. Mayo Clin Proc 1997; 72:871–878.

3. Weinshenker BG. Epidemiology of multiple sclerosis. Neurol Clin 1996; 14:291–308.

4. Kurtzke JF, Wallin MT. Epidemiology. In: Burks JS, Johnson KP, eds. Multiple sclerosis diagnosis, medical management and rehabilitation. New York: Demos, 2001.

5. Kurtzke JF. Epidemiology of multiple sclerosis. In: Vinken PJ, Bruyn GW, Klawans HL, eds. Handbook of clinical neurology, vol 3, no 47. Amsterdam: Elsevier; 1985: 259–287.

6. Ebers G, Kukay K, Bulman D, et al. A full genome search in multiple sclerosis. Nat Genet 1996; 13:472–476.

7. Sadovnick A, Ebers G, Dyment D, et al. Evidence for genetic basis of multiple sclerosis. Lancet 1996; 347:1728–1730.

8. Poser CM. Viking voyages: the origin of multiple sclerosis? An essay in medical history. Acta Neurol Scand 1995; 161(suppl):11–22.

9. Hammond SR, deWytt C, Maxwell LC, et al. The epidemiology of multiple sclerosis in the three Australian cities: Perth, Newcastle, and Hobart. Brain 1988; 111:1–25.

10. Hammond S, DeWytt CMD, et al. The epidemiology of multiple sclerosis in Queensland, Australia. J Neurol Sci 1987; 80:185–204.

11. Ebers G, Sadovnick AD. The geographic distribution of multiple sclerosis: a review. Neuroepidemiology 1993; 12:1–5.

12. Dean G, Grimaldi G, Kelly R, et al. Multiple sclerosis in southern Europe I: Prevalence in Sicily in 1975. J Epidemiol Community Health 1979; 33:107–110.

13. Vassallo L, Elian M, Dean G. Multiple sclerosis in southern Europe II. Prevalence in Malta in 1978. J Epidemiol Community Health 1979; 33:111–113.

14. Dean G. Annual incidence, prevalence, and mortality of multiple sclerosis in white South-African-

born and in white immigrants to South Africa. Br Med J 1967; 2:724–730.

15. Kurtzke JF, Dean G, Botha DPJ. A method of estimating age at immigration of white immigrants to South Africa, with an example of its importance. S Afr Med J 1970; 44:663–669.

16. Alter M, Leibowitz U, Speer J. Risk of multiple sclerosis related to age at immigration to Israel. Arch Neurol 1966; 15:234–237.

17. Detels R, Visscher RM, Malmgren B, et al. Evidence for lower susceptibility to multiple sclerosis in Japanese-Americans. Am J Epidemiol 1977; 105:303–310.

18. Alter M, Okihiro M, Rowley W, et al. Multiple sclerosis among Orientals and Caucasians in Hawaii. Neurology 1971; 21:122–130.

19. Kurtzke JF, Hyllested K. Multiple sclerosis in the Faroe Islands. I. Clinical and epidemiological features. Ann Neurol 1979; 5:6–21.

20. Kurtzke JF, Hyllested K. Multiple sclerosis in the Faroe Islands II. Clinical update, transmission, and the nature of MS. Neurology 1985; 36:307–328.

21. Kurtzke JF, Hyllested K. Multiple sclerosis in the Faroe Islands III. An alternative assessment of the three epidemics. Acta Neurol Scand 1987; 76:317–339.

22. Kurtzke JF, Hyllested K, Heltberg A. Multiple sclerosis in the Faroe Islands: transmission across four epidemics. Acta Neurol Scand 1995; 91:321–325.

23. Kurtzke JF, Gudmundsson KR, Bergmann S. Multiple sclerosis in Iceland: I. Evidence of a postwar epidemic. Neurology 1982; 32:143–150.

24. Rosati G, Aiello I, Granieri E, et al. Incidence of multiple sclerosis in the town of Sassari, Sardinia, 1965–1985: evidence for increasing occurrence of the disease. Neurology 1988; 38:384–388.

25. Gronning M, Riise T, Kvale G, et al. Incidence of multiple sclerosis in Hordaland, Western Norway: a fluctuating pattern. Neuroepidemiology 1991; 10:53–61.

26. Gronning M, Mellgren SI. Multiple sclerosis in the two northernmost counties of Norway. Acta Neurol Scand 1985; 72:321–327.

27. Poser CM, Paty DW, Scheinberg L, et al. New diagnostic criteria for multiple sclerosis: guidelines for research protocols. Ann Neurol 1983; 13:227–231.

28. Duquette P, Murray TJ, Pleines J, et al. Multiple sclerosis in childhood: clinical profile in 125 patients. J Pediatr 1987; 111:359–363.

29. Gilden DH, Devlin ME, Burgoon MP, Owens GP. The search for virus in multiple sclerosis brain. Mult Scler 1996; 4:179–183.

30. Cook SD, Dowling PC, Russell WC. Multiple sclerosis and canine distemper. Lancet 1978; i:605–606.

31. Cook SD, Natelson BH, Levin BE, Chavis PS, Dowling PC. Further evidence of a possible association between house dogs and multiple sclerosis. Ann Neurol 1978; 3:141–143.

32. Ross RT. The varicella-zoster virus and multiple sclerosis. J Clin Epidemiol 1998; 51:533–535.

33. Knox KK, Brewer JH, Henry JM, Harrington DJ, Carrigan DR. Human herpesvirus 6 and multiple sclerosis: systemic active infections in patients with early disease. Clin Infect Dis 2000; 31:894–903.

34. Sriram S, Mitchell W, Stratton C. Multiple sclerosis associated with *Chlamydia pneumoniae* infection of the CNS. Neurology 1998; 50:571–572.

35. Sriram S, Mitchell W, Stratton C. Multiple sclerosis associated with *Chlamydia pneumoniae* infection

of the CNS. Neurology 1998; 50:571–572.

36. Sriram S, Stratton CW, Yao S, et al. *Chlamydia pneumoniae* infection of the central nervous system in multiple sclerosis. Ann Neurol 1999; 46:6–14.

37. Panitch HS. Influence of infection on exacerbations of multiple sclerosis. Ann Neurol 1994; 36:S25–S28.

38. Siva A, Radhakrishnan K, Kurland LT, O'Brien PC, Swanson JW, Rodriguez M. Trauma and multiple sclerosis: a population-based cohort study from Olmsted County, Minnesota. Neurology 1993; 43:1878–1882.

39. Banford CR, Sibley WA, Thies C, et al. Trauma as an etiologic and aggravating factor in multiple sclerosis. Neurology 1981; 31:1229–1234.

40. Goodin DS, Ebers GC, Johnson KP, et al. The relationship of MS to physical trauma and psychological stress. Report of the Therapeutics and Technology Assessment Subcommittee of the American Academy of Neurology. Neurology 1999; 52:1737–1745.

41. Confavreux C, Hutchinson M, Hours MM, Cortinovis-Tourniaire P, Moreau T. Rate of pregnancy-related relapse in multiple sclerosis. Pregnancy in Multiple Sclerosis Group. N Engl J Med 1998; 339:285–291.

42. Ebers GC Bulmon DE, Sadovnick AD et al. A population-based study of multiple sclerosis in twins. N Engl J Med 1986; 315:1638–1642.

43. Sadovnick A, Baird P, Ward R. Multiple sclerosis: updated risks for relatives. Am J Med Genet 1988; 29:533–541.

44. Ebers GC, Sadovnick AD, Risch NJ. A genetic basis for familial aggregation in multiple sclerosis. Canadian Collaborative Study Group. Nature 1995; 377:150–151.

45. Gaudet JP, Hashimoto L, Sadovnick AD, Ebers GC. Is sporadic MS caused by an infection of adolescence and early adulthood? A case-control study of birth order position. Acta Neurol Scand 1995; 91:19–21.

46. Ebers GC, Sadovnick AD. Susceptibility: genetics in multiple sclerosis. In: Paty DW, Ebers GC, eds. Multiple sclerosis. Philadelphia: FA Davis; 1998: 29–47.

4
Diagnosis and differential diagnosis

Overview

In this era of MS disease-modifying therapies there is increased emphasis on early accurate diagnosis. No single test is crucial, and diagnosis is generally based on a suggestive history and neurological examination, consistent demographic profile, and supportive laboratory data. Although clinical criteria alone can be sufficient, most patients undergo selected paraclinical tests to exclude other conditions and optimize confidence that the diagnosis is correct. Certain general diagnostic principles provide helpful guides (Table 4.1).

This chapter will begin with a review of formal diagnostic criteria for MS, then consider the clinical and laboratory aspects of diagnosis, clinical variants which can mimic MS, clues to misdiagnosis, and the differential diagnosis of MS.

Table 4.1 General MS diagnostic principles.

- Diagnosis has multiple direct benefits for the patient:
  - to remove diagnostic uncertainty
  - to identify candidates for therapy
  - to guide selection of disease modifying therapy
  - to provide a prognosis and allow informed planning
  - to produce an improved sense of well being
- Common as well as unusual conditions can mimic MS
- The misdiagnosis rate of 5–10% involves overdiagnosis most often based on improper interpretation of brain MRI lesions
- There are also problems with underdiagnosis
- Clinical diagnosis should be supported by laboratory data, to minimize misdiagnosis and to clarify the prognostic profile
- Blood tests are useful to rule out alternative diagnoses and co-diagnoses
- MRI and CSF are the key laboratory tests; their sensitivity increases over time
- Other laboratory tests are ancillary

Formal diagnostic criteria

Although formal diagnostic criteria for MS date back to 1954,[1] in 1965 Schumacher outlined basic clinical principles that are still followed today [2] (Table 4.2). The Schumacher criteria acknowledged MS as a white matter disease which affected young people from 10 to 50 years of age, and which could take a relapsing or progressive course. Relapses had to last at least 24 hours, while the slow worsening that constituted progression had to be observed for a minimum of 6 months. The core concept was evidence of lesions disseminated in time and space. The criteria made no formal reference to paraclinical evaluation, but implicit to the requirement of no better explanation was formulation of a differential diagnosis, and exclusion of other conditions.

Subsequent advances in neuroimaging, cerebrospinal fluid (CSF) analysis, and electrophysiologic studies led to recognition that these paraclinical tests showed patterns of abnormalities associated with MS. Although Bauer was the first to publish criteria which incorporated laboratory tests,[3] the 1983 Poser Committee criteria became the main diagnostic reference for MS (Table 4.3).[4] They have been used in particular for research protocols. The Poser criteria recognized definite and probable MS diagnostic categories,which could be clinically or laboratory supported. The acceptable age for disease onset was increased to 59 years. The definition of a relapse was expanded to include brief symptoms such as Lhermitte sign or paroxysmal attacks, provided they recurred multiple times over a period of days to weeks. Relapses could be historic, without medical corroboration. Clinical evidence required documented abnormalities on examination, which could include historic documentation from medical records. A laboratory-supported diagnosis required abnormal CSF, either IgG oligoclonal bands (OCB) or intrathecal IgG production. The Poser criteria contain some confusing aspects, and appear to allow a laboratory-supported definite diagnosis with a single clinical attack. There were subsequent clarifications that suggested that a diagnosis of primary progressive MS,

Table 4.2 Diagnosis based on Schumacher criteria.[2]

- Appropriate age (10–50 years)
- CNS white matter disease
- Lesions disseminated in time and space
- Objective abnormalities
- Consistent time course
  - attacks lasting >24 hours, spaced 1 month apart
  - slow/stepwise progression for >6 months
- No better explanation
- Diagnosis by a competent clinician (preferably a neurologist)

Table 4.3 Poser Committee criteria.[4]

Category	Attacks	Clinical evidence		Paraclinical evidence	CSF
Clinical diagnosis					
Definite	2	2	or	–	
	2	1	or	1	
Probable	2	1	or	–	
	1	2	or	–	
	1	1	or	1	
Laboratory-supported diagnosis					
Definite	2	1	or	1	+
	1	2	or	–	+
	1	1	or	1	+
Probable	2	–	or	–	+

which was in essence a single attack, would require a distinct new event or lesion. Such patients might have to be observed for two or more years before that requirement was met. In relapsing patients at a first attack, other clinical or paraclinical evidence had to develop at a later and clearly distinct timepoint to count as a second attack.[5]

The most recent review of diagnostic criteria for MS took place at a meeting in London in July 2000.[6] The goal of this International Panel on the Diagnosis of MS, a consortium put together by MS societies in Europe and North America, was to create simplified diagnostic criteria for the practicing physician that could also be adopted for research protocols. Definitions were to be clarified, new information on MRI was to be incorporated into diagnosis (including MRI requirements for dissemination in time and space), and the diagnosis of primary progressive MS was to be addressed. The International Panel reaffirmed that there had to be objective evidence of dissemination in time and space. An attack was defined as a neurological disturbance, lasting 24 or more hours, that was clearly distinguishable from an infection or metabolic related pseudoattack. An attack could also consist of multiple paroxysmal events, occurring over one or more days. Two attacks had to be separated by a minimum of 30 days between onset. These new diagnostic criteria recognize definite MS, possible MS, or not MS categories. The only incorporated paraclinical tests are MRI, CSF, and visual evoked potentials (VEPs). CSF parameters include a recommendation to use more sensitive techniques to detect OCB (Table 4.4). MRI criteria are specified to determine dissemination in time and space. Dissemination in space is adopted from studies of Barkhof and Tintoré, and require that three of four criteria be met: (1) nine T2 hyperintense brain lesions, or one contrast enhancing lesion; (2) at least one infratentorial lesion; (3) at least one juxtacortical lesion; (4) at least three

Table 4.4 Recommended CSF abnormalities to use in the diagnosis of MS.[6]

- IgG OCB bands distinct from serum
  - isoelectric focusing the prefered technique
- Elevated IgG index
- Less than 50 mononuclear WBC/mm³

periventricular lesions.[7,8] MRI lesions should be at least 3mm in size, and one spinal cord lesion may substitute for a brain lesion. Criteria for dissemination in time depend on when the initial brain MRI is done (Table 4.5).

These revised diagnostic criteria rely heavily on MRI (Table 4.6). They do not allow a definite diagnosis to be made at the time of a first attack, unlike other recently proposed diagnostic criteria.[9] CSF is incorporated when MRI lesions are fewer in number than required. The diagnosis of definite primary progressive MS requires MRI and CSF abnormalities, as well as either clinical progression over one year or MRI dissemination in time (see Chapter 7).[10] Abnormal VEP reduces the number of MRI lesions required. The panel also acknowledged the broad differential diagnosis of MS, and included cerebrovascular disorders, collagen vascular diseases, infections, paraneoplastic syndromes, and monophasic or recurrent demyelinating disease variants.[6] These recommended diagnostic criteria were designed for specificity rather than sensitivity. Modifications are being considered to simplify the criteria and improve their sensitivity.

Clinical diagnosis

The fact that MS has a characteristic demographic profile is helpful (Table 4.7). Most patients are Caucasian women of child-bearing age. With regard to age, MS rarely begins before age 10 or after age 60. Childhood MS shows a female predominance, with frequent brainstem involvement at onset. In a recent series of 1826 consecutively evaluated patients, 0.8%

Table 4.5 MRI criteria for dissemination in time.

When first MRI is 3 or more months after clinical event
A single contrast lesion (at an independent site) documents dissemination in time
If there are no contrast lesions, a second MRI is done (recommended interval at 3 months); a new T2 or contrast lesion documents dissemination in time

When first MRI is within 3 months of clinical events, a second MRI is done at least 3 months after clinical event
A single contrast lesion documents dissemination in time
If there are no contrast lesions, a third MRI is done at least 3 months after the first scan; a new T2 or contrast lesion documents dissemination in time

Table 4.6 Suggested new diagnostic criteria for MS.[6]

Clinical presentation	Space	Time
Two or more attacks; objective clinical evidence of two or more lesions	Not required	Not required
Two or more attacks; objective clinical evidence of one lesion	Abnormal MRI or Two or more MRI lesions + abnormal CSF or New attack at new site	Not required
One attack; objective clinical evidence of two or more lesions	Not required	MRI criteria met or Second attack
One attack; objective clinical evidence of one lesion (first attack patients)	MRI criteria met or Two or more MRI lesions + abnormal CSF	MRI criteria met or Second attack

Table 4.7 Demographic profile of MS.

- Female gender preference
  - Overall MS is 70–75% female
  - Female predominance in all clinical subtypes except primary progressive (gender ratio 1 : 1)

- Young adult
  - Onset between ages 15 and 50 in 90% of MS patients
  - Average age of onset 28–30
  - Fewer than 1% have onset before age 10 or over age 60
  - Adolescent onset (before age 16) in 1.2–6%

- Racial preference
  - Greater than 90% Caucasian
  - Unusual in Asians, Afro-Americans
  - Unknown or rare in Africans, Eskimos, Native Americans, Inuits, Hutterites, Maoris, Aboriginals

- Geographic
  - Low, medium, high risk zones
  - Increased in temperate vs. tropical climates

had onset of MS at age 60 or older. All but one were primary progressive, with a female predominance of 87%.[11] Progressive myelopathy was a common presentation. With regard to race, MS is virtually unknown in Africans, Eskimos, and native Americans, and rare in Asians. Afro-

Americans show an intermediate frequency between Caucasians and Africans. Disease features may be influenced by race, presumably on a genetic basis. MS tends to be more severe in Afro-Americans, while Asians often show a clinical syndrome of spinal cord-optic nerve disease, similar to Devic's neuromyelitis optica.[12] Patients with this so-called Asian type MS show an older age at disease onset, have fewer brain MRI lesions, more enhancing spinal cord lesions, and have distinct human leukocyte antigen (HLA) haplotype associations. With regard to geography, MS is mainly a temperate zone disease.

MS shows distinct clinical patterns which have been divided into subtypes by expert consensus (Table 4.8).[13] Most patients begin with relapsing disease, and only a minority (15%) show a progressive course from onset. Patients with a slow worsening from onset (either primary progressive or progressive relapsing subtype) appear similar, so that the occurrence of occasional superimposed relapses may not be a meaningful distinguishing factor.[14] This progressive group shows an equal gender ratio, has an older age of onset (>35 years of age), and often presents with a progressive myelopathy syndrome.

Most MS patients start out with a relapsing-remitting course, characterized by acute neurological attacks (also called relapses, exacerbations, flareups) separated by periods of clinical stability. Attacks most often involve motor, sensory, cerebellar, and visual systems (Table 4.9). As disease duration increases, cognitive, sexual, and sphincter involvement become more common. Among relapsing patients, about 5–10% seem to

Table 4.8 MS clinical subtypes.

Subtype	Frequency	Clinical course
Relapsing	85% of initial cases 55% of all MS	Acute attacks, with clinical stability between attacks
Primary progressive	10%	Slow worsening from onset; never experiences acute attacks
Progressive relapsing	5%	Slow worsening from onset, with subsequent superimposed acute attacks
Secondary progressive	Ultimately 90% of untreated relapsing MS; 30% of all MS	Relapsing patients with transition to slow worsening, with or without superimposed acute attacks

Table 4.9 Characteristic MS clinical relapses.

- Motor abnormalities (weakness, spasticity)
- Sensory disturbances (numbness, paresthesias, pain, Lhermitte sign)
- Cerebellar abnormalities (incoordination, imbalance, tremor)
- Vision disturbances (monocular decrease in vision and color perception, with eye pain)
- Brainstem abnormalities (diplopia, trigeminal neuralgia, internuclear ophthalmoplegia)
- Bladder difficulties (urgency, frequency, overflow leakage, incontinence, inability to void)
- Bowel difficulties (constipation, rarely diarrhea, fecal incontinence)
- Sexual dysfunction
- Cognitive difficulty

have benign disease characterized by mild attacks, excellent recovery, and no appreciable disability even years into the disease. Such patients are said to have benign MS, but this is a retrospective diagnosis, and there are no uniformly accepted criteria.

Although progressive patients generally slowly worsen without recovery, they can remain clinically stable for up to several years, and may even show short term minor improvements.[15]

From a clinical viewpoint then, MS should be considered in any young person who presents with CNS abnormalities that spontaneously remit, particularly in a Caucasian female. Certain clinical syndromes highly suggest MS (Table 4.10). In addition, MS should be considered in older individuals (particularly males) who present with a slowly progressive spinal cord syndrome.

Table 4.10 Clinical syndromes which highly suggest MS in a young individual.

- Unilateral optic neuritis
- Incomplete transverse myelitis
- Internuclear ophthalmoplegia
- Isolated brainstem or cerebellar syndrome
- Multifocal CNS white matter syndrome
- Trigeminal neuralgia
- Lhermitte's sign
- Paroxysmal neurological attacks (brief, stereotypic, repetitive)
- Neurological syndrome associated with heat sensitivity, excessive fatigue

Laboratory diagnosis

Although a number of paraclinical tests can be helpful to make the diagnosis of MS and exclude other conditions, the primary laboratory tests are blood studies, MRI, and to a more limited extent CSF analysis (Table 4.11). The appropriate selection of tests depends on the final differential diagnosis, formulated after a thorough history and examination.

Table 4.11 Paraclinical tests used in the diagnosis of MS.

Primary tests
- Blood work
  - Excludes alternative diagnosis, co-diagnosis
  - Brain MRI with or without contrast
  - Spinal cord MRI with or without contrast
- Cerebrospinal fluid analysis

Secondary tests
- Evoked potentials (EPs)
  - Visual EP most useful
  - Somatosensory EP (lower extremities)
- Urodynamics (to document neurogenic bladder)
  - Bladder ultrasound (post void residual)
  - Cystometrogram
- Neurocognitive tests
- Autonomic tests
  - Sympathetic skin responses

Other
- Biopsy
  - Skin
  - Node
  - Brain/leptomeninges
  - Other sites (lacrimal/lip/salivary glands, etc.)
- Angiography
  - Cerebral
  - Fluorescein
  - MR angiography
- Electrophysiologic
  - Nerve conduction tests
  - Electromyography
- Chest X-ray
  - Hilar adenopathy
- Miscellaneous
  - Schirmer test
  - Salivary gland scintigraphy
  - Brain SPECT
  - Kveim test
  - Gallium scan

Primary laboratory tests

Blood studies are useful to exclude many disorders in the differential diagnosis of MS (Table 4.12). The appropriate selection of tests depends on the final differential diagnosis, formulated after a thorough history and examination.

MRI is the key diagnostic test for MS. It generally shows brain lesions in a highly suggestive pattern. MRI also has prognostic value. The role of MRI for diagnosis of MS is discussed in detail in Chapter 7. Briefly, contrast brain MRI is done unless there is a contraindication. Spinal MRI is reserved

Table 4.12 Blood studies that can be useful in the diagnostic workup for MS.

Tests	Alternative diagnosis
ANA, anti-dsDNA, anti-ribonucleoproteins (Ro/SS-A, La/SS-B, U1) and related autoantibodies, cryoglobulins	Collagen vascular disease (systemic lupus erythematosus, Sjögren syndrome, mixed connective tissue disease, systemic sclerosis)
Anticardiolipin antibodies	Antiphospholipid syndrome
Antibodies to viruses (retroviruses, herpes viruses, and others), to spirochetes (*B. burgdorferi, T. pallidum*), and other bacteria (*Chlamydia pneumoniae, Brucella* species); polymerase chain reaction for selected agents	Infection (tropical spastic paraparesis, HTLV-I associated myelopathy, AIDS, viral encephalomyelitis, Lyme disease, syphilis, brucellosis, *Chlamydia* encephalomyelitis)
Endocrine studies (thyroid function tests, glucose, cortisol)	Thyroid disease, hypoglycemia, Addison's disease
Vitamin studies (vitamins B_{12} and E; homocysteine, methylmalonic acid; folate)	Vitamin deficiency syndrome
Angiotensin converting enzyme, IgG, calcium	Neurosarcoidosis
Sedimentation rate, C reactive protein, ANCA	Vasculitis
Very long chain fatty acids	Adrenoleukodystrophy, adrenomyeloneuropathy
Mitochondrial DNA mutations	Mitochondrial cytopathies (Leber, adult onset Leigh disease, Kearns–Sayre, MELAS, MERRF)
Antineuronal antibodies	Paraneoplastic syndromes
Anti-acetylcholine receptor antibodies	Myasthenia gravis
Blood smear	Acanthocytosis
Gene testing	Genetic disorders

for older individuals (above age 50), those with a spinal cord presentation, those in whom it is important to rule out spinal cord pathology, or individuals who have a normal or atypical brain MRI.

CSF analysis is safe although somewhat more invasive than neuroimaging. It can provide unique complementary information about intrathecal immune abnormalities. In first attack patients, abnormal CSF has predictive value for MS. In certain circumstances CSF analysis is a mandatory part of the workup (Table 4.13). As noted in the diagnostic criteria discussion, the most important CSF tests are OCB, followed by intrathecal IgG production (Table 4.14).[16] Although OCB have high specificity for MS, they can be seen in any chronic infectious or inflammatory CNS disorders. Paired blood and CSF samples must be run, since OCB which leak from blood into CSF do not indicate intrathecal immune disturbance. Sometimes a single monoclonal band is reported. This may reflect a transitional state which will evolve into OCB. Although not normal, a monoclonal band does not have the same diagnostic significance as OCB. Another CSF test, myelin basic protein (MBP), is not

Table 4.13 Indications for CSF analysis in the diagnostic workup for MS.

- Suspected primary progressive MS
- Normal/atypical MRI
- Atypical clinical presentation

Table 4.14 CSF tests in MS.

- OCB
  - Most specific CSF test
  - Isoelectric focusing preferred to agarose gel electrophoresis (improved sensitivity)
  - Must be run as paired (CSF, blood) samples correlates with plasma cell infiltration of meninges
  - Initially positive in 60–65% of patients, ultimately positive in 90–95%
  - Once positive bands stay positive
  - False positive rate 4–9% (higher in infectious/inflammatory disorders)

- Intrathecal IgG production
  - Either IgG index, or 24 hour production
  - Run as paired sample
  - Initially positive in 60–65% of patients, ultimately positive in 70–90%
  - Once elevated test stays positive
  - False positive rate increases at high and low CSF protein levels

- Myelin basic protein
  - Nonspecific marker of CNS tissue damage (low specificity)
  - Values fluctuate in MS
  - Variable sensitivity (assay dependent)

very useful. Levels fluctuate over time, and any process which damages CNS tissue can produce a positive value. This CSF test does not have high sensitivity or specificity for MS.

The sensitivity of both MRI and CSF to detect abnormalities in MS increases over time, so that it is rare years into the disease to have both nonsupportive MRI and CSF.

Secondary laboratory tests

A variety of other diagnostic tests may also be useful (Table 4.11). Evoked potential tests are used to document lesion dissemination in space, to provide objective evidence for a subjective complaint, or to confirm a pattern of CNS involvement consistent with MS. They are not needed when a clinical diagnosis of MS is supported by consistent MRI and/or CSF findings. Latency prolongation is more helpful than decreased amplitude and wave dispersion, since it suggests a demyelinating process. With visual EPs, a latency of greater than 10 milliseconds between the eyes is abnormal even when the absolute values are within normal range. However, factors such as drowsiness, inattention, inability to focus, or visual problems can all impair responses. For somatosensory EPs, lower extremity testing is more valuable than upper extremity testing since it evaluates the entire spinal cord. Brainstem auditory EPs are less helpful than visual or somatosensory EPs, and are not recommended.[17] Autonomic nervous system abnormalities are present in a proportion of MS patients, and this can be tested.[18,19] For example, the addition of sympathetic skin responses increases the yield for electrodiagnostic abnormalities by 14%.[20]

In unusual circumstances a number of other diagnostic procedures may be indicated for MS. Additional ancillary laboratory testing might include urodynamics to document neurogenic bladder, neurocognitive tests to document cognitive abnormalities, nerve conduction tests to rule out peripheral nerve involvement, or skin biopsy to diagnose cerebral autosomal dominant arteriopathy with subcortical infarctions and leukoencephalopathy (CADASIL).[21,22]

Clinical variants

There are disorders which involve CNS white matter, have an inflammatory component, and mimic features of MS.[23] They are all currently considered to be in the clinical spectrum of MS (Table 4.15). Some are likely to be true variants or form-frustes of MS, while others show fundamental differences.

Table 4.15 Clinical variants of MS.

- Monophasic syndromes
  - Postinfectious encephalitis/encephalomyelitis
  - Clinically isolated syndromes (optic neuritis, transverse myelitis/myelopathy, isolated brainstem/cerebellar syndrome) and multifocal syndromes
- Devic's neuromyelitis optica
- Marburg variant MS
- Unilateral mass lesion (tumefactive MS)
- Balo's concentric sclerosis
- Myelinoclastic diffuse sclerosis (Schilder disease)
- Disseminated subpial demyelination

Monophasic syndromes

Postinfectious encephalitis/acute disseminated encephalomyelitis

Postinfectious encephalitis is a monophasic syndrome which typically follows infection or vaccination.[24–28] It is also called postinfectious encephalomyelitis and acute disseminated encephalomyelitis (ADEM), since both brain and spinal cord are often affected. Part of the spectrum of ADEM involves a more severe and hyperacute syndrome, acute hemorrhagic necrotizing encephalomyelitis (AHNE). ADEM is estimated to account for up to 20% of acute encephalitis cases. It does not reflect direct infection of the CNS, but rather immune-mediated damage initiated by a prior triggering event. Most cases involve a single attack, but self-limited recurrent episodes (often multiple, in a similar brain territory) have been reported to occur over months.[29–32]

A number of triggering events are associated with ADEM, although viral infections are the most common (Table 4.16). For many years exanthematous infections (particularly measles) were the most common triggering pathogens. One in 1000 cases of measles infection developed ADEM. With effective vaccine programs for measles, vaccinia, and rubella, such cases have dropped precipitously. Nonspecific respiratory pathogens are now the most commonly implicated group of viruses.[33]

Although there are no absolute criteria, classic ADEM has a number of features which differentiate it from MS (Table 4.17).[34–39] Brain MRI abnormalities can be quite dramatic (Figure 4.1).

ADEM is most common in children and adolescents, but can occur in adults. In a recent series of adults initially diagnosed as ADEM, 35% had a subsequent event that led to a diagnostic reclassification as MS.[40] Basic characteristics that showed a significant correlation with ADEM as opposed to MS were older age, prior infection, and shorter duration of symptoms before admission. The only significant difference in initial clinical symptoms was a higher frequency of brainstem problems in ADEM patients (16% vs. 3%). Fever, loss of consciousness, and meningismus were only seen with ADEM. ADEM patients were significantly more likely to show an elevated CSF albumin quotient (indicating damage to the blood–CSF barrier), and to show infratentorial MRI lesions. In contrast to this adult series, where multifocal first attack MS patients were likely to have been unrecognized, in a recent pediatric series only 14% with an initial diagnosis of ADEM were reclassified as MS.[41] Children may present

Table 4.16 Triggering events associated with ADEM.

Infection
- Viruses
  - Coxsackie B
  - Hepatitis A, B
  - Herpes agents (cytomegalovirus, Epstein–Barr virus, human herpes virus type
       6, herpes simplex virus, varicella zoster virus)
  - Measles
  - Mumps
  - Retroviruses (human immunodeficiency virus, human T cell lymphotrophic
       virus type 1)
  - Rubella
  - Upper respiratory tract pathogens (influenza A and B, respiratory syncytial
       virus)
- Other pathogens
  - *Bordetella pertussis*
  - *Borrelia burgdorferi*
  - Campylobacter
  - Chlamydia
  - Cryptococcus
  - Legionella
  - Malaria
  - *Mycoplasma pneumoniae*
  - *Rickettsia rickettsiae*
  - *Salmonella typhi*
  - Streptococci

Vaccination
- Diptheria–tetanus–pertussis
- Hog virus
- Influenza
- Japanese B encephalitis
- Measles
- Rabies
- Smallpox
- Typhus

Serum treatments

Drugs
- Gold
- Streptomycin

Unknown

with prominent ataxia, cranial nerve palsies, and hemiparesis. Another study evaluated children with monophasic ADEM ($n = 28$), relapsing ADEM (7), or MS[42] (2000). In contrast to MS, the ADEM group was characterized by prior infection, polyregional presentation, corticospinal tract involvement, encephalopathy, and bilateral optic neuritis. Unilateral optic neuritis occurred only in MS, while seizures occurred only in ADEM. ADEM patients showed peripheral leukocytosis, CSF pleocytosis, and elevated CSF protein, while MS patients showed CSF OCB. MRI confirmed that periventricular lesions were uncommon in the ADEM group, and that most children showed clearance or improvement of lesions on subsequent study, without new lesions.

ADEM has no documented treatment. A number of modalities are reported to be helpful, and glucocorticoids are commonly used as first line therapy (Table 4.18).[43-46] Supportive care is critical, since patients typically do very well once over the acute illness.

AHNE is a hyperacute, fulminant illness which typically follows influenza or nonspecific respiratory infection.[47,48] It shows a number of differences from ADEM, but there are examples of patients with ADEM who develop the more severe form (Table 4.19). Patients with AHNE present with a syndrome that mimics an expanding mass lesion. They can show marked peripheral leukocytosis (up to 30,000 WBC), and an elevated erythrocyte

Table 4.17 Features which distinguish ADEM from MS.

- Basic features
  - Monophasic event (rare cases are relapsing or chronic)
  - Identifiable preceding event (infection, vaccination) in 70%
  - Onset is abrupt
  - Most cases in the pediatric or very young adult age range
  - No gender preference
  - Characteristic clinical syndrome is a severe encephalopathy with multifocal involvement (depressed level of consciousness, seizures, bilateral optic neuritis, complete transverse myelitis with areflexia)
  - Unusual presentations can mimic brain tumor, psychosis
  - Mortality rate of up to 20% (the more severe cases)
- MRI features
  - Lesions tend to be bilateral, extensive, and somewhat symmetric
  - Many lesions enhance
  - Periventricular lesions are relatively uncommon
  - Lesions may show mass effect
  - Asymptomatic basal ganglia lesions are relatively common (up to 40%)
  - Followup MRI shows resolution of lesions (up to 33%), or partial lesion resolution without new lesions (at least 67%)
- CSF features
  - Moderate pleocytosis is common
  - OCB and intrathecal IgG production are uncommon
  - If present, OCB and increased intrathecal IgG production are transient

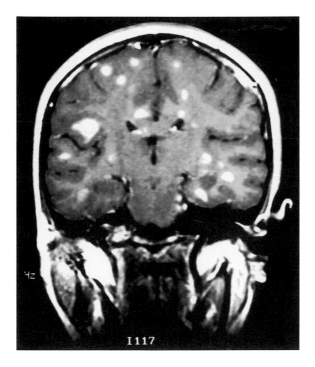

Figure 4.1
Coronal image from the brain MRI of a patient with ADEM showing multiple
contrast-enhanced lesions.

sedimentation rate (ESR). CSF pleocytosis can be as high as 3000 WBC
per mm³, with a mixed or neutrophilic predominance, as well as RBCs. The
pathology of AHNE involves widespread necrosis of small blood vessels,
intense inflammatory response, and multiple small hemorrhages superimposed on the perivenular demyelination that is typical of ADEM.
Neuroimaging can show massive cerebral lesions, with general, focal, or
even unilateral involvement. AHNE has a higher mortality rate than ADEM,
with death typically within the first week. Although survivors can be left with
permanent deficits, they can also show excellent recovery despite prolonged coma.

Table 4.18 Treatments used for postinfectious encephalitis.

- Glucocorticoids
- Adrenocorticotropin
- Intravenous immune globulin
- Plasma exchange
- Cyclophosphamide
- Glatiramer acetate
- Polyinosine-polycytidylic acid-polylysine stabilized with carboxymethylcellulose

Table 4.19 Features that distinguish ADEM from AHNE.

Feature	ADEM	AHNE
Typical age	Children	Young adults
Trigger	Exanthematous viruses	Influenza, respiratory tract viruses
Course	Acute	Hyperacute, fulminant
CSF	Mononuclear pleocytosis	Neutrophilic pleocytosis, RBCs
Neuroimaging	White matter lesions	Large cerebral lesions
Pathology inflammation,	Perivenular inflammation with demyelination	Blood vessel necrosis, multiple small hemorrhages superimposed on demyelination

Clinically isolated syndromes

Certain syndromes which affect a single region of the CNS can be post-infectious, or can be the first attack of MS.[49,50] Examples are isolated optic neuritis, incomplete transverse myelitis, and isolated brainstem or cerebellar syndromes. They are referred to as clinically isolated syndromes (CISs). The first attack of MS can also be a multifocal syndrome, very similar to ADEM but without typical encephalopathy and increased intracranial pressure symptoms. Patients with unifocal and multifocal monophasic syndromes may never develop MS. Normal brain MRI and CSF predict very low risk for the development of MS over the next several years, while abnormalities on brain MRI or CSF consistent with MS predict high risk (in the range of 80–90%) for the development of MS. In fact, quantitative measurement of initial brain MRI lesion load and number predict subsequent clinical status and MRI activity (reviewed in Chapter 7). Optic neuritis is the first MS attack in 8–33% of cases, part of a multifocal first attack in 24–41% of cases, and ultimately occurs in 27–66% of all MS patients. The risk of development of MS after an isolated optic neuritis has been reported to range from 12–85%, but over time is at least 75%. The risk of MS steadily rises during the first 2 to 5 years following optic neuritis, but then increases more gradually. Risk factors for MS after optic neuritis have been identified (Table 4.20).[51] In contrast to adolescents and adults, children (under age 10) rarely go on to develop MS.[52]

Acute transverse myelitis can also occur as a first attack of MS (myelopathic MS), or as an isolated event. Complete transverse myelitis carries low risk for MS (2–8%), while incomplete transection carries a much higher risk (72–80%). Abnormalities on brain MRI (59–93%), CSF (78%), or evoked potentials (EPs) (30%) consistent with MS all increase the positive predictive value for MS over the next few years. Features against a diagnosis of MS are symmetric motor and sensory findings, a swollen spinal cord on MRI, or large multilevel spinal cord confluent lesions on MRI.

Table 4.20 Factors related to risk of development of MS after acute optic neuritis.

↑ *Risk*
- Young adult (26–40)
- Venous sheathing
- Recurrent optic neuritis
- Female sex
- History of minor neurologic symptoms
- Brain MRI lesions
- CSF OCB or intrathecal IgG production

↓ *Risk*
- Age < 10
- Macular star/exudates
- Retinal or disc hemorrhage
- Severe disc edema
- No brain MRI lesions
- Normal CSF

Neuromyelitis optica

Neuromyelitis optica (Devic's disease) is a syndrome which involves lesions affecting the optic nerve (typically bilateral) and spinal cord.[53-55] Involvement of these two anatomic regions occurs within a restricted time frame. This can range from simultaneous onset, to onset within a period of several years. At the current time there are no uniformly accepted criteria for the diagnosis of Devic's neuromyelitis optica, although the Mayo Clinic has suggested specific clinical and laboratory criteria (Table 4.21).[56,57]

Table 4.21 Proposed diagnostic criteria for neuromyelitis optica.[57]

- Absolute criteria
  - Optic neuritis
  - Acute myelitis
  - No evidence of clinical disease outside the optic nerve, spinal cord

- Major supportive criteria
  - Initial brain MRI negative
  - Spinal cord MRI lesion extending over three or more segments
  - CSF pleocytosis >50 WBC per mm^3 or >5 neutrophils per mm^3

- Minor supportive criteria
  - Bilateral optic neuritis
  - Severe optic neuritis (fixed deficit > 20/200 vision in at least one eye)
  - Severe fixed deficit in motor function of at least one limb (MRC grade ≤ 2/5)

*Patient must meet all absolute criteria, and either one major or two minor supportive criteria.

Only 10% of Devic's neuromyelitis optica patients appear to have classic MS. The rest have a disorder which seems quite different (Table 4.22).[58-62] The cause of Devic's neuromyelitis optica is unknown. It appears to be more common in Asians, who often show an optic nerve–spinal cord form of MS. Non-MS Devic's neuromyelitis optica takes two distinct courses. It is either monophasic (35%) or relapsing (55%). The monophasic form affects both genders, and shows a younger age at onset (mean onset 27 years). Most patients make a reasonable recovery, although occasional individuals have a relentlessly progressive course to death. The relapsing form is more frequent in women (by almost 4 : 1), is associated with a worse overall outcome, and is characterized by frequent and severe relapses. Respiratory failure occurs in 22% of cases.

Spinal MRI is markedly abnormal in Devic's neuromyelitis optica, with changes over multiple segments (Figure 4.2). There may be abnormalities involving most of the spinal cord. By contrast, brain MRI is often entirely normal, although in the relapsing form brain lesions ultimately occur in half of patients.

Children with Devic's neuromyelitis optica have a much better prognosis than adults, and most make an excellent recovery.[63] Although treatment is not established, glucocorticoids and azathioprine are reported to be helpful.[64-66] Intravenous immune globulin and plasma exchange have also been used.[67] Cyclosphosphamide, methotrexate, and interferon β seem to be ineffective.

The etiology of Devic's neuromyelitis optica is unknown, and may involve different factors. Patients appear to show an immunopathology involving deposition of antibody and complement within areas of active demyelination, and there may be many granulocytes and eosinophils. The topographic distribution of spinal cord and optic nerve involvement is similar to that seen in experimental disease involving autoantibodies directed against myelin oligodendrocyte glycoprotein (MOG), a CNS myelin antigen. This antigen is currently under study.[68]

Acute Marburg variant

MS may take an acute fulminant course without remission, leading to death within a year. This has been referred to as acute Marburg type/variant MS.[69-73] There are not many well studied cases in the literature. The course is generally monophasic and rapidly progressive, with death from brainstem involvement. Most cases occur in young people without any prior neurological history, although a few patients with documented MS have gone on to a fulminant and terminal course. Pathological changes include widespread demyelination, axon loss, edema, macrophage infiltration, and presence of granulocytes and eosinophils. Some, but not all patients, show acute plaque pathology involving deposition of immunoglobulin and complement.

It can be difficult to differentiate Marburg variant from ADEM, especially when the time course involves weeks. Autopsy studies on a single patient

Table 4.22 Features which differentiate Devic's neuromyelitis optica and MS.

Feature	Neuromyelitis optica	MS
Clinical course	Relapsing (55%) or monophasic (35%); 10% have MS	No monophasic course, relapsing (85% at onset) or progressive
Therapeutic response	Responds to glucocorticoids, azathioprine	Responds to disease modifying therapy (interferon beta, glatiramer acetate, mitoxantrone)
MRI	Normal brain MRI	Abnormal brain MRI ($\leq$ 95%)
	Abnormal spinal MRI ($\leq$ 100%) Acute diffuse swelling	Abnormal spinal MRI ($\leq$ 75%) Scattered peripheral lesions
	Three or more spinal segments involved Optic chiasm signal changes	Less than two spinal segments involved Optic nerve signal changes
CSF	Pleocytosis common	Pleocytosis uncommon ($\leq$ 33%)
	> 100 WBC/mm^3 Neutrophil predominance	< 50 WBC/mm^3 Mononuclear predominance
	$\uparrow$ Protein common; > 150 mg/dl (41%) $\uparrow$ CSF/serum albumin quotient OCB, intrathecal IgG production rare	$\uparrow$ Protein uncommon; < 100 mg/dl Normal CSF/serum albumin quotient OCB ($\leq$ 95%), intrathecal IgG production (70–90%) common
	$\downarrow$ Matrix metalloproteinases (MMP-9)	$\uparrow$ Matrix metalloproteinases (MMP-9)
Blood studies	$\uparrow$ Sedimentation rate (33%) $\downarrow$ HLA-DR2 $\uparrow$ Autoantibodies ANA ($\leq$ 50%)	Normal sedimentation rate $\uparrow$ HLA-DR2 No marked autoantibody association
Pathology	Necrosis, vascular proliferation, variable perivascular inflammation	Perivenular demyelinated plaques

with Marburg variant found pronounced post-translational MBP changes, which converted mature MBP to an extensively citrullinated and poorly phosphorylated immature form.[74] It has been postulated that such changes could make myelin more susceptible to breakdown.

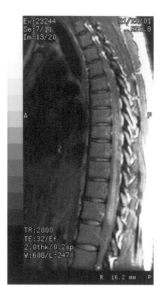

Figure 4.2
A T2 weighted image of the thoracic spinal cord shows a lesion with
hyperintense signal typical of Devic's disease.

Unilateral mass lesion (tumefactive MS)

Most MS lesions are less than 2 cm in diameter.[75] However, occasionally
plaques show ring enhancement, surrounding edema, and mass effect, to
mimic brain tumor or abscess. This can occur in patients with established
MS and otherwise typical lesions, or can occur at presentation.[76-80] There
are also patients with a tumefactive demyelinating lesion and disease
features atypical for MS, but similar to ADEM.[81] Helpful neuroimaging features to distinguish plaque from tumor include reduced regional cerebral
blood flow on perfusion MRI, evidence for increased diffusion, and
decreased magnetization transfer.

Balo's concentric sclerosis

Balo's concentric sclerosis is a rare acute variant of MS with a characteristic pathology.[82-91] Large concentric bands of demyelination are separated
by bands of intact myelin, to give an expanding ring appearance. Recent
immunopathology studies have linked this disorder to a pathology of distal
dying back oligodendrogliopathy with oligodendrocyte apoptosis, the so-
called Pattern III acute plaque pathology.[92] The clinical course is quite
severe. Illness starts acutely, with progression over weeks to months.
Patients may die within a year from increased intracranial pressure and
cerebral herniation, or from systemic complications such as pneumonia.
Sometimes the course is subacute, and rare patients may survive years.
Most cases are between the ages of 20 and 50 years, but can be as young

as 4 years of age. Patients present with an increased intracranial pressure syndrome and cerebral symptoms (headache, depressed level of consciousness, seizures, aphasia, cognitive loss). Balo's concentric sclerosis may be more common in the Philippines and China than in other parts of the world. The diagnosis is suggested by an MRI pattern of unusual ring-like lesions.[93-98] CSF may show OCB and intrathecal IgG production. In the pre-MRI era diagnosis was made at autopsy. Treatment has included glucocorticoids, immunosuppressives, and plasma exchange with immunoabsorption. It can be difficult to distinguish Balo's concentric sclerosis from acute Marburg variant MS (see above), apart from the distinctive pathology. To further confuse the picture, there are examples of patients with concentric lesions and typical MS plaques. In contrast to MS, classic typical Balo's concentric sclerosis is confined to the cortex without significant lesions in the spinal cord, cerebellum, brainstem, or optic chiasm.

Myelinoclastic diffuse sclerosis
Myelinoclastic diffuse sclerosis is also called Schilder disease or childhood MS.[99-103] Initial reports misdiagnosed cases of adrenoleukodystrophy and subacute sclerosing panencephalitis, so that true myelinoclastic diffuse sclerosis is extremely rare with only a handful of documented cases. Myelinoclastic diffuse sclerosis is a pediatric disorder characterized by bilateral symmetric, very large (3 by 2 cm) hemispheric lesions. The lesions are predominantly demyelinating, but may also involve axon damage, tissue necrosis, and subsequent cavitation. Subcortical U fibers can be involved in addition to adjacent cortex. Children often present with visual problems (such as cortical blindness), seizures, headache, and vomiting. Some pathology studies report a mononuclear cell inflammation maximal in the demyelinated areas rather than the peripheral rim of the active lesion, which suggests that the immune response could be secondary to myelin breakdown. Glucocorticoids have been used as treatment.[104] The disorder is so rare that it has been questioned as a true disease entity.

Disseminated subpial demyelination
Two cases of demyelination localized to the subpial region have been described.[105,106] They both had loss of myelin with relative axon pairing. One patient showed marked inflammatory changes, while the other showed minimal infiltrates. Both patients had focal neurological deficits accompanied by a change in mental status that would be considered unusual for MS.

Clues to misdiagnosis

An estimated 5–10% of MS patients are misdiagnosed.[107] Certain scenarios increase the risk of misdiagnosis (Table 4.23).[108] Since many diseases produce lesions on brain MRI which can mimic MS (Figure 4.3), it is important not to base a diagnosis solely on MRI findings.[109,110] The occurrence of certain clinical features should suggest that a patient may not have MS, and this is more likely as the number of atypical features rises (Table 4.24). There are also atypical MRI (Table 4.25) and CSF features (Table 4.26) that should raise the possibility of a misdiagnosis.

Table 4.23 Scenarios that lead to misdiagnosis of MS.

- Make the diagnosis without any laboratory tests
- Diagnose MS despite a normal neurological examination
- Do not consider the possibility of a genetic disorder
- Diagnose MS despite normal CSF and normal or atypical brain MRI
- Make the diagnosis despite atypical features

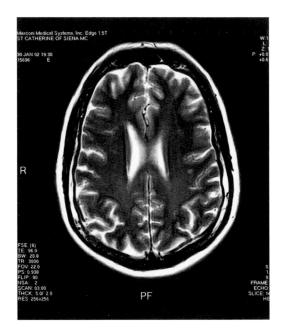

Figure 4.3
A T2 weighted image from a patient with Lyme disease showing white matter lesions that may lead to a misdiagnosis of MS. This is only one example of many conditions in which MRI may mimic MS.

Differential diagnosis

The differential diagnosis of MS is extensive because the disease is so variable (Table 4.27).[5] Although most conditions are excluded after a thoughtful history and examination, it is important to at least consider these alternative disease categories in the initial patient assessment.

Table 4.24 Clinical clues for MS misdiagnosis.

- Normal examination
- Lack of dissemination in time and space
- Onset before age 10 or after age 55
- Progressive subtype starting before age 35
- Localized disease
- Extraneural disease
- Atypical clinical features
  - Impaired level of consciousness
  - Prominent fever, uveitis, headache, or pain (except trigeminal neuralgia)
  - Abrupt hemiparesis or hearing loss
  - No abnormalities of optic nerve, eye movements, sensation or bladder
  - Peripheral neuropathy
  - Nonscotomatous field defects
  - Progressive myelopathy without bladder or bowel involvement
  - Gray matter features (prominent early dementia, seizures, aphasia, fasciculations, extrapyramidal features)

Table 4.25 MRI clues for MS misdiagnosis.

- Brain
  - Normal brain MRI
  - Very small lesions
  - Subcortical lesion localization (such as internal capsule)
  - Predominant infratentorial involvement
  - Prominent gray matter involvement (such as basal ganglia)
  - Symmetric, confluent hemispheric white matter involvement
  - Significant mass effect
  - Hydrocephalus
  - Focal cerebellar, brainstem atrophy
  - Absence of callosal or periventricular lesions
- Spinal cord
  - Lesion > 2 vertebral segments long
  - Severe swelling
  - Full thickness lesions

Table 4.26 CSF clues for MS misdiagnosis.

- Normal CSF
- Disappearance of OCB
- Normalization of intrathecal IgG production
- Cell count > 50 WBC /mm^3
- Protein > 100 mg/dl; ↑ CSF albumin quotient

Genetic

Multiple inherited disorders can mimic MS (Table 4.28).[111] Although there are rare families where multiple members have MS, only 20% of patients report a relative with the disease, and a strongly positive family history is

(MERRF). Clinical manifestations generally involve neurological and muscle dysfunction. Leber disease involves acute or subacute vision loss with bilateral optic atrophy. Although young men between adolescence and age 30 are most often involved, women and older males can also be affected. Additional features can include ataxia, atrophy, weakness, spasticity, dysarthria, hyperreflexia, sensory loss, and dystonia. Leber disease most commonly involves mutations in mitochondrial DNA coding for subunits of complex I (NADH hydrogenase). About 50% of cases are due to a single mutation in the fourth subunit. Other (sometimes multiple) mutations involve complex I, III and IV genes. Diagnosis is confirmed by gene testing, and suggested by a positive family history, ophthalmologic examination, and abnormalities on electrocardiogram and visual EPs. Subacute necrotizing encephalomyelopathy (Leigh syndrome) involves progressive spongiosis and necrosis of brainstem, midbrain, and basal ganglia.[114] Typical onset is in infancy or childhood, but occasionally there are adult onset cases. Patients develop decreased vision, dysarthria, ataxia, seizures, dementia, and myoclonus. Leigh syndrome is genetically heterogeneous, with both AR recessive and X-linked inheritance, and can involve nuclear or mitochondrial genes. Defects include cytochrome oxidase deficiency, pyruvate dehydrogenase complex defects, mutations in the mitochondrial gene coding for ATPase 6, and respiratory chain and complex I deficiency. All these defects affect terminal oxidative metabolism with impaired energy production. Diagnosis involves mitochondrial DNA analysis, plasma amino acid analysis, ophthalmologic examination, brain MRI, urinary organic acid analysis, and measurement of muscle or fibroblast pyruvate dehydrogenase, pyruvate carboxylase, cytochrome c oxidase, and complex I. MELAS is a genetically heterogeneous disorder that involves in most cases a mutation in the mitochondrial gene coding the tRNA for leucine. The classic picture is that of stroke-like episodes in young adults which can resemble relapsing MS. Other features include hearing loss, recurrent headaches, vomiting, optic atrophy, seizures, and cognitive loss. Diagnosis involves analysis of mitochondrial DNA, blood and CSF lactate and pyruvate, plasma alanine, ophthalmologic examination, brain MRI, and urinary organic acid analysis. Lactic acidosis is variable and can be mild; it is most likely to be elevated during acute episodes. MERRF in most cases is due to a mutation in the mitochondrial gene encoding the tRNA for lysine. The classic syndrome involves myoclonus, seizures, myopathy, and cerebellar ataxia. Other features can include cardiomyopathy, hearing loss, optic atrophy, fatigue, spasticity, peripheral nervous system (PNS) disease, and dementia. The spectrum ranges from a rapidly progressive full blown syndrome to clinically asymptomatic. Diagnosis can be made by DNA analysis, and can be supported by: elevated CPK, lactate, and pyruvate; muscle biopsy; EEG, EKG, nerve conduction studies, and visual evoked potentials; ophthalmologic and hearing evaluations.

In addition to the genetic vitamin E deficiency noted above, there are genetic disorders of other vitamins. Most genetic forms of cobalamin (vitamin B_{12}) deficiency present under age one. However, cobalamin G mutation and plasma R binder (transcobalamin I) deficiency can occur during adulthood. Neurological abnormalities include paresthesias, position and vibration loss, ataxia, spasticity, and weakness. Hematologic abnormalities include macrocytic anemia, neutrophilic hypersegmentation, and megaloblastic bone marrow changes. Diagnostic workup for this vitamin deficiency includes cobalamin, methionine, and homocysteine levels; hematocrit, mean red blood cell volume, peripheral blood smear; and Schilling test. Methylenetetrahydrofolate reductase deficiency, a genetic folate deficiency, can present in late childhood and adulthood with progressive spasticity and hyperreflexia (particularly involving lower extremities), incoordination, fatigue, paresthesias, and diplopia. Patients do not show megaloblastic anemia, and serum folate may be only slightly reduced. Methionine and homocysteine are very useful screening tests, and a specific enzyme assay is available.

The organic acidemia which is most likely to masquerade as MS is biotinidase deficiency, which can present with intermittent ataxia, optic atrophy, and occasionally white matter lesions on brain MRI. Diagnosis involves demonstration of elevated levels of the organic acid 3-hydroxy-isovaleric acid.

The peroxisomal disorders which mimic MS are X-linked adrenoleukodystrophy (ALD) and adrenomyeloneuropathy (Table 4.30).[115,116] They present (in older children and adults respectively) with progressive neurological syndromes. ALD produces cognitive problems, incoordination, and visual/auditory disturbances. Adrenomyeloneuropathy presents with worsening myelopathy and mild polyneuropathy. Episodic vomiting, bronzed

Table 4.30 Adrenoleukodystrophy (ALD).

- Involves mutations in the gene encoding ALD protein (Xq28)
- Several male phenotypes
  - Childhood cerebral (48%), adolescent cerebral (5%), adult cerebral (3%) forms
  - Adrenomyeloneuropathy (25%)
  - Addison disease only (asymptomatic, presymptomatic) (8%)
- Female phenotype
  - 10–15% of heterozygous women develop adrenomyeloneuropathy symptoms (3rd–5th decades)
- Children show visual and cerebral features; adults show slowly progressive spinal cord syndrome
- MRI lesions show predilection for parieto-occipital white matter
- CSF is normal
- Diagnosis based on plasma very long chain fatty acids

skin, adrenal insufficiency, and polyneuropathy are suggestive features. Very long chain fatty acids in plasma are diagnostic.

Wilson's disease is an AR condition with abnormal copper metabolism.[117,118] Copper is deposited in liver, brain, kidney, and cornea. Neurological presentations typically occur between ages 20 and 40, with dysarthria, incoordination, and involuntary movements. Subsequently pseudobulbar palsy, cognitive loss, and behavioral abnormalities are seen. MS is most likely to be misdiagnosed in the setting of a prominent cerebellar syndrome. Diagnosis involves slit lamp examination for Kayser–Fleischer rings and sunflower cataracts; serum copper and ceruloplasmin; and 24 hour urinary copper excretion.

Infectious

CNS infections can produce syndromes similar to MS (Table 4.31). Human herpes virus type 6 (HHV-6) is a neuroinvasive and CD4+ T cell tropic agent. It causes exanthem subitum (roseola) in childhood, and has been associated with unusual examples of focal CNS demyelinating disease (encephalitis and myelopathy) in both immunocompetent and immunocompromised hosts. Serology, polymerase chain reaction (PCR), culture, and immunostaining are used to document active infection. Several laboratories are investigating the possibility that HHV-6 is an etiologic factor in a subset of MS patients,[119,120] Varicella zoster virus (VZV) is another herpes virus which produces a leukoencephalitis involving white matter, but only in immunocompromised hosts.

Measles virus on rare occasions (one per million population) causes a slow virus infection which can be confused with MS in children and adolescents. It causes neurological problems, abnormal brain MRI, and CSF immune disturbances. Subacute sclerosing panencephalitis (SSPE) typically involves children and adolescents, but has occurred as late as age 32. Cases are seen in countries which do not have measles immunoprophylaxis programs. Atypical features for MS include early behavioral or personality changes, progressive dementia, and late myoclonus. CSF has

---

Table 4.31 Differential diagnosis of MS: infectious syndromes.

- Viruses
  - Herpes virus infection
  - Measles (subacute sclerosing panencephalitis)
  - Retroviruses (HTLV-1, HIV)
  - JC virus (progressive multifocal leukoencephalopathy)
- Bacteria
  - *Brucella* species
  - *Chlamydia pneumoniae*
  - Spirochetes (Lyme disease, syphilis)

oligoclonal bands and intrathecal IgG production, but there are markedly elevated antibody titers to measles in both CSF and serum.

Progressive multifocal leukoencephalopathy (PML) is a slow virus infection due to JC virus, a ubiquitous papovavirus.[121] PML involves progressive demyelination in patients with impaired cellular immunity. It occurs in 4% of HIV-I infected individuals, as well as in the setting of intensive immunosuppressive therapy. PML produces characteristic worsening MRI lesions which may occur in the hemisphere, brainstem, cerebellum, and even corpus callosum. Lesions do not enhance, show no associated edema, and most often involve parieto-occipital subcortical regions. They have a scalloped appearance to follow the gray–white interface. Features which are atypical for MS involve visual field cuts, cortical blindness, cognitive loss, and personality changes. CSF is usually normal, but occasionally shows mild pleocytosis or protein elevation. Patients progess to death within months. Brain biopsy provides a definitive diagnosis, but PCR of CSF, brain tissue, or peripheral lymphocytes can confirm the presence of viral DNA.

Two retroviruses must be considered in the differential diagnosis of MS. The AIDS virus, human immunodeficiency virus type I (HIV-I), causes meningitis, encephalopathy, and myelopathy. There are rare cases associated with relapsing and remitting neurological disease virtually indistinguishable from MS, referred to as HIV-I associated leuko-encephalomyelopathy.[122–124] CNS lesions contain retrovirus. This MS-like syndrome generally occurs with initial infection, but it has preceded infection manifestations by several years. Patients typically experience intermittent disease attacks, but occasionally the course is more fulminant and ends in death within weeks. Brain MRI shows white matter lesions, and CSF shows increased IgG levels and detectable myelin basic protein. It is not clear whether these patients have two distinct diagnoses, or whether in rare cases HIV-1 can produce a demyelinating CNS disease similar to MS. Human T cell lymphotropic virus type I (HTLV-I), the first identified human retrovirus, is a type C oncovirus which is particularly prevalent in southern Japan (20% infection rate) and in the Caribbean (2–5% infection rate). Virus is transmitted by sexual contact, blood transfusion, from mother to child, or through use of contaminated needles. Approximately 1% of infected individuals develop a progressive spinal cord disease, tropical spastic paraparesis/HTLV-1 associated myelopathy (TSP/HAM).[125] TSP/HAM mimics progressive MS. The typical age of onset is 35–45, and women are affected three times as often as men. The lower thoracic cord is preferentially involved, and motor features outweigh sensory features. Patients show a progressive spastic paraparesis with impotence, neurogenic bladder, and dysesthesias out of proportion to objective sensory loss. They have specific antibodies to HTLV-I in blood and CSF, with intrathecal production. Half of patients show nonperiventricular MRI lesions. Spinal MRI shows swelling with enhancement early, and atrophy late. TSP/HAM is probably an immune mediated process since there is tissue infiltration by CD4+ and CD8+ T cells initially, followed by predominantly cytotoxic CD8+ cells. Blood T cells show marked spontaneous proliferation.

Chlamydia pneumoniae is an obligate intracellular pathogen which is implicated in atherosclerotic disease. In rare cases this bacterial agent can cause meningitis and encephalitis, and has been implicated in MS based largely on CSF polymerase chain reaction and antibody data, as well as reported reactivity with OCB.[126]

Brucellosis is a worldwide zoonotic infection (particularly prevalent in the Mediterranean and Middle East) due to *Brucella melitensis* and several other species.[127] Infection involves exposure to animals, raw milk, infected cheese or cream products, or infected aerosols. Some 2–5% of patients develop neurological involvement. Encephalomyelitis is a rare neurological syndrome, which can be associated with MRI white matter lesions and CSF oligoclonal bands. Diagnosis is suggested by a history of exposure, CSF pleocyctosis with elevated protein, and positive serology.

Spirochetal infections such as Lyme disease and syphilis can mimic MS. Lyme disease is due to the tick-borne spirochete *Borrelia burgdorferi*.[128] Early dissemination can be associated with cranial neuropathy. The facial nerve is often involved, but Lyme disease can rarely produce optic neuropathy, as well as oculomotor and trigeminal nerve syndromes. These early neurological syndromes frequently follow or are coincident with erythema migrans, a pathognomonic expanding red rash at the tick bite site. Even without antibiotics, it spontaneously remits. Late stage infection is rarely associated with an encephalomyelitis that can produce brain and spinal cord syndromes which mimic MS. Patients slowly worsen without treatment. Features which help to differentiate neurological Lyme disease from MS include: prior or concurrent extraneural disease (skin, musculoskeletal, cardiac, or ocular disease); multisystem complaints (fatigue, headache, stiff neck, arthralgias, myalgias, palpitations); prior or concurrent peripheral nervous system involvement; blood and CSF seropositivity to *B. burgdorferi*, particularly intrathecal organism-specific antibody production; significant mononuclear pleocytosis with elevated protein; and (in North American Lyme disease) absence of CSF oligoclonal bands or intrathecal nonspecific IgG production.

Syphilis is due to the spirochete *Treponema pallidum*. Neurosyphilis syndromes which mimic MS include meningovascular syphilis and parenchymatous neurosyphilis. Meningovascular syphilis, a vasculitis of small and medium sized blood vessels, typically occurs 5–7 years after infection. Patients experience prodromal symptoms including vertigo or behavioral changes over weeks to months, followed by acute focal neurological deficits particularly involving the middle cerebral artery. CSF shows mononuclear pleocytosis, elevated protein, and reactive VDRL; the workup makes it clear that CNS blood vessels are the primary target. Parenchymatous neurosyphilis (general paresis and tabes dorsalis) occurs years after initial infection. General paresis presents with slowly worsening cognitive or psychiatric features, with subsequent focal neurological deficits (tremor, dysarthria, incontinence). Tabes dorsalis affects the lower spinal cord with lightning pains or paresthesias, proprioceptive loss, wide based gait, and incontinence. Optic atrophy, oculomotor problems, and pupil disturbance (Argyl Robertson pupil) can also be seen. In tabes dorsalis, in particular, CSF changes are not marked, but VDRL is generally positive.

Inflammatory

Certain inflammatory disorders can masquerade as MS (Table 4.32). Behçet disease is a multisystem inflammatory disorder of young adults which involves the CNS in 5–25% of patients.[129–132] Males generally show a more severe disease course. Although neuro-Behçet shows similarities to MS and can take a relapsing or progressive course, it is also quite different (Table 4.33). Suggestive features include corticospinal tract and brainstem involvement, intracranial hypertension, and mental status changes. Sensory, visual, and cerebellar features are less common. Patients develop recurrent oral and genital ulcerations, uveitis, and pathergy. Neurological involvement involves vasculitic changes particularly affecting the upper brainstem, basal ganglia, internal capsules, and peduncles. In acute disease, large confluent brainstem lesions extending into the basal ganglia and diencephalon are highly suggestive. Brainstem atrophy occurs in 21%. In chronic disease cerebral white matter lesions can be seen. Unlike MS, lesions are numerous in nonperiventricular as well as periventricular areas. Among the collagen vascular diseases, systemic lupus erythematosus (SLE), mixed connective tissue disease, systemic sclerosis, and Sjögren's disease can mimic MS.[133,134] They all show suggestive extraneural involvement and autoantibody patterns. Neurological involvement occurs in up to 75% of SLE patients, including transverse myelitis and optic neuritis. Sjögren disease can also produce transverse myelitis and optic neuropathy. In a recent study, 17% of patients with a diagnosis of primary progressive MS met criteria for Sjögren disease.[135] SLE tends to produce subcortical, cortical and deep gray matter lesions on MRI, in contrast to those seen in MS. Helpful differentiating features are

Table 4.32 Differential diagnosis of MS: inflammatory disorders.

- Behçet disease
- Collagen vascular disease (systemic lupus erythematosus, mixed connective tissue disease, systemic sclerosis, Sjögren's disease)
- Myasthenia gravis
- Neurosarcoidosis

suggestive extraneural disease (skin and kidney involvement, anemia, thrombocytopenia, Sicca syndrome, systemic symptoms) and diagnostic autoantibodies (to nuclear antigens, double stranded DNA, ribosomal antigens). Myasthenia gravis can present in young women with waxing and waning abnormalities that can raise the question of MS. Attacks are short and tend to come with physical effort, or later in the day. Approximately 5% of patients with sarcoidosis have neurological involvement, both CNS and peripheral nervous system (PNS).[136,137] Brain MRI can show periventricular white matter lesions, but additional findings of meningeal enhancement,

Table 4.33 Comparison of neuro-Behçet disease and MS.

	Neuro-Behçet	MS
Age of onset	Young adults	Young adults
Gender preference	Male	Female
Disease course	Relapsing, progressive	Relapsing, progressive
Extraneural involvement	Present	Absent
Clinical features	Fever common Predominantly or exclusively motor ↑ intracranial pressure in 11–35% Spinal cord involvement uncommon	Fever unusual Sensory as well as motor involvement common Normal intracranial pressure Spinal cord involvement common
Disease activity	↓ with age	Persists with age
Prognostic features	Early onset unfavorable	Early onset favorable
Lesion location	Upper brainstem, basal ganglia, internal capsule, peduncles Large vessels often involved Cortex and cerebellar lesions unusual	Cortex, subcortex, periventricular white matter, optic nerves, brainstem, cerebellum No vascular involvement
CSF	Pleocytosis (often neutrophilic), ↑ protein common Intrathecal IgG production OCB uncommon and may disappear	Pleocytosis, ↑ protein unusual Intrathecal IgG production OCB common and remain positive
MRI	Abnormal in 50% Brainstem lesions extend into the basal ganglia, diencephalon Brainstem atrophy (late)	Abnormal in 90–95% Periventricular, centrum semiovale, and corpus callosum lesions

hydrocephalus, or enhancing mass lesions suggest an alternative diagnosis. Although neurological involvement may be the presenting feature of sarcoidosis, it more commonly develops in a patient with known disease. Suggestive features are ocular involvement, diabetes insipidus from hypothalamic involvement, hilar adenopathy, anergy, abnormal chest X-ray, positive gallinium scan, increased calcium and total IgG, and CSF pleocytosis.

Metabolic

Certain metabolic disorders can be mistaken for MS (Table 4.34). Cobalamin deficiency causes pernicious anemia.[138] Associated neurological problems are subacute combined degeneration, optic neuropathy,

Table 4.34 Differential diagnosis of MS: metabolic disorders.

- Cobalamin deficiency
- Folate deficiency
- Vitamin E deficiency

peripheral neuropathy, and cognitive loss. Subacute combined degeneration produces paresthesias, vibration and position loss, and spastic paraparesis. Suggestive features include symmetric involvement, macrocytic anemia, gastric achlorhydria, hypersegmented neutrophils, megaloblastic bone marrow, low vitamin B_{12} levels, high metabolite (homocysteine, methylmalonic acid) levels, and positive Schilling test. MRI can show scattered white matter lesions, but CSF is generally normal. Folate deficiency has been noted in some cases of subacute combined degeneration; patient symptoms improve after replacement therapy. Acquired vitamin E deficiency, which can result from intestinal fat malabsorption as a sequelae of surgical resection or hepatobiliary disease, can produce spinocerebellar abnormalities with a polyneuropathy.[139,140] Treatment involves vitamin E supplementation.

Miscellaneous

There are several miscellaneous conditions which produce features similar to MS (Table 4.35). Chronic fatigue syndrome (CFS) is defined by the Centers for Disease Control and Prevention as a syndrome of unexplained persistent or relapsing fatigue.[141,142] Patients must have four or more additional symptoms (memory/concentration problems, myalgias, arthralgias, sleep disturbance, headache, prolonged postexertional fatigue, sore throat, tender lymph nodes). Although fatigue is prominent in MS, CFS patients rarely have objective neurological features, and MRI/CSF studies do not suggest MS.

Table 4.35 Differential diagnosis of MS: miscellaneous conditions.

- Chronic fatigue syndrome
- Complicated migraine conditions
- Idiopathic central serous choroidopathy
- Leukoencephalopathy with vanishing white matter
- Migratory sensory neuritis
- Neuroretinitis (optic disc edema with macular star)
- Peripheral nerve, root, plexus conditions
- Sporadic system degeneration
- Systemic histiocytosis

Table 4.36 Features of central serous choroidopathy.

- Male to female ratio 6–10 : 1
- Typical onset age 20–55, type A personality
- Acute monocular vision loss
- Serous retinal detachment, with abnormal fluorescein/indocyanine green
  angiography

Central serous choroidopathy is a condition which is more common in men. It produces monocular vision loss that can mimic optic neuritis; the serous detachment can be quite subtle (Table 4.36). This MS masquerader emphasizes the importance of a complete (dilated) fundus examination in all patients who present with monocular vision loss.

Migratory sensory neuritis produces paresthesias or pain sensations over various body parts. Any objective sensory loss is in a peripheral nerve distribution, and MRI/CSF studies are normal.

Neuroretinitis is an anterior optic neuritis (papillitis) characterized by a macular exudate, or so called "macular star".[143] Although patients range from 8 to 50 years of age, most are in the third or fourth decade. Up to half of patients report an upper respiratory tract infection in the preceding one to two weeks, followed by monocular vision impairment. The exudates reflect a disc vasculopathy, with secondary leakage of lipoproteinaceous material into the macular.

PNS syndromes occasionally mimic MS. Sporadic system degenerations also occur. Systemic histiocytosis, a reticuloendothelial system disorder involving fever, pancytopenia, and hepatosplenomegaly, occasionally produces CNS lesions.[144] Unusual neurological features are diabetes insipidus and PNS involvement. MRI lesions show sustained enhancement. CSF shows elevated protein and albumin index, rather than OCB and intrathecal IgG production.

Neoplastic

Among neoplastic disorders in the differential diagnosis of MS (Table 4.37), lymphoma (particularly the intravascular form, neoplastic angio-endotheliomatosis) can produce multifocal neurological deficits with brain MRI lesions that can mimic MS. Although there may be a temporary gluco-corticoid response, the course is typically inexorably downhill and can mimic acute fulminant (Marburg variant) MS. Patients often show elevated ESR, skin lesions, and systemic symptoms.

Paraneoplastic syndromes may occur in patients before their malignancy is realized. Patients may show CSF oligoclonal bands, pleocytosis, increased protein, and intrathecal IgG production. A variety of antineuronal antibodies are associated with paraneoplastic disease.

Table 4.37 Differential diagnosis of MS: neoplastic disorders.

- Intravascular lymphoma (neoplastic angioendotheliomatosis)
- Metastatic tumor
- Primary brain tumor
- Paraneoplastic syndrome

Psychiatric

Although somatiform disorders can manifest as episodic neurological problems, and patients with anxiety, panic, and hyperventilation attacks can experience paresthesias and even transient focal features, such patients have normal or inconsistent examinations, subjective complaints, and normal CSF and MRI studies, or MRI studies with fixed deficits. This is a diagnosis of exclusion (Table 4.38).

Table 4.38 Differential diagnosis of MS: psychiatric disorders.

- Anxiety disorder
- Conversion disorder
- Depression

Structural

Vascular malformations, disk disease, cervical spondylosis, arachnoiditis, and congenital conditions (Arnold–Chiari malformation, syrinx, arachnoid cyst) can produce MS-like symptoms (Table 4.39). Lesions in the foramen magnum region, brainstem, or upper spinal cord produce multiple abnormalities. Appropriate neuroimaging detects most such lesions, which do not produce CSF immune disturbances. Both arachnoid cysts (particularly

Table 4.39 Differential diagnosis of MS: structural conditions.

- Arachnoid cyst
- Arachnoiditis
- Arnold–Chiari malformation
- Cervical spondylosis
- Spinal cord disk disease
- Syrinx
- Vascular malformation

in the cisterna magna region) and spinal cord cysts can cause episodic deficits. Late onset Chiari malformations can produce cerebellar ataxia, spastic paraparesis, nystagmus, Lhermitte's sign, and trigeminal neuralgia. In contrast to MS there is neck and upper extremity pain, and nystagmus is often vertical.

Brainstem and spinal cord vascular malformations in particular can mimic fluctuating deficits of MS. Spinal cord dural arteriovenous fistulas and true arteriovenous malformations produce venous hypertension, with resultant edema, ischemia, and tissue damage. The results are a thoracic myelopathy which can be acute, relapsing, or progressive.[145] Spinal cord MRI shows patchy intramedullary increased signal. Myelography (prone and supine) may show vermiform filling defects due to dilated draining veins, but selective spinal angiography remains the definitive diagnostic test. Treatment involves angiographic embolization, surgical repair, or radiosurgery.

Toxic (Table 4.40)

Nitrous oxide exposure can produce progressive myeloneuropathy with prominent sensory disturbances.[146] There may be optic nerve involvement as well. Exposure to nitrous oxide anesthesia (e.g. during dental treatment) should suggest the diagnosis. Nitrous oxide inactivates cobalamin, so that features are similar to B_{12} deficiency.

Osmotic myelinolysis, or central pontine myelinolysis (CPM), is a demyelinating disorder of the ventral pons which occurs with extreme

Table 4.40 Differential diagnosis of MS: toxic disorders.

- Nitrous oxide toxicity
- Osmotic myelinosis (central pontine myelinolysis)
- Postchemotherapy leukoencephalopathy
- Radiation injury
- Subacute myelo-optic neuritis (clioquinol toxicity)
- Trichloroethylene poisoning

serum hyperosmolality, rapid correction of hyponatremia, and possibly nutritional factors. Up to 10% of cases have extrapontine myelinolysis, usually involving cerebellum.

Chemotherapy agents such as ciclosporin (cyclosporin), tacrolimus (FK506), and methotrexate can produce focal white matter abnormalities, and cytosine arabinoside and 5-fluorouracil can produce cerebellar syndromes.[147] The temporal relationship to drug exposure is a key diagnostic clue.

Radiation can produce a transient myelopathy 3–6 months after exposure, characterized by Lhermitte sign or paresthesias. A late progressive myelopathy occurs in 2–3% of irradiated patients, particularly those who received hyperthermia. Radiation can injure brain tissue, ranging from demyelination to coagulation necrosis, and can present as a mass lesion months to years after the radiation exposure.

Clioquinol is used to treat traveller's diarrhea and chronic gastroenteritis. It can be neurotoxic, and produces a syndrome called subacute myelo-opticoneuropathy.[148,149] Spinal cord and optic nerves are affected. Gastrointestinal symptoms are followed by ascending numbness and weakness with bowel and bladder involvement, autonomic abnormalities, prominent paresthesias, and subsequent vision loss.

Trichloroethylene is an organic solvent. It can cause cranial neuropathies (of the trigeminal, facial, optic, and oculomotor nerves), and rarely bulbar, cerebellar, and extrapyramidal problems. The diagnosis is suggested by associated peripheral nerve damage, and exposure to toxic fumes.

Vascular

Vascular disease can produce focal CNS deficits mimicking MS (Table 4.41). Antiphospholipid antibody syndrome is associated with antibodies to cardiolipin and lupus anticoagulant, and can occur in healthy individuals, or in association with SLE, infection, neoplasm, or drug exposure.[150,151] Clues to this masquerader are a history of thrombosis, fetal loss, and other SLE or related symptoms (livedo reticularis, photosensitivity, arthritis, sicca

Table 4.41 Differential diagnosis of MS: vascular conditions.

- Antiphospholipid syndrome
- CADASIL
- Eale disease
- Hypertensive cerebrovascular disease
- Multiple cerebral emboli
- Periventricular leukomalacia
- Retrocochlear vasculopathy of Susac
- Subcortical arteriosclerotic leukoencephalopathy (Binswanger)
- Vascular headache (migraine)
- Vasculitis

syndrome) (Table 4.42). Neuroimaging lesions in this disorder involve the superficial and deep territory of major cerebral arteries.

CADASIL is an arteriopathy involving the notch 3 gene (Table 4.43).[152-157] Gene carriers develop progressive brain MRI lesions, even in the asymptomatic stage. Ultimately there is rather symmetric white matter and basal ganglia involvement with bilateral confluent lesions. Fronto-orbital and occipital subcortical areas are relatively spared, in contrast to MS. Patient develops transient ischemic attacks, followed by repeated strokes and ultimately dementia despite the absence of vascular risk factors. CSF is normal, and there is no cranial nerve or spinal cord involvement.

Table 4.42 Antiphospholipid syndrome (APS).

Suggestive history
   Thrombotic episodes
   History of fetal loss
   Other antiphospholipid syndrome/systemic lupus erythematosus
      related symptoms

Suggestive laboratory abnormalities
   Anticardiolipin antibodies
   MRI (putamenal lesions vs. white matter, posterior fossa)

Indicated therapy
   Anticoagulation

Table 4.43 Features of CADASIL.

- AD condition involving notch 3 gene mutation (19p13.1)

- Suggestive clinical picture
   - Recurrent ischemic episodes (TIA, CVA) in 71% (gait disturbance develops in 90%, urinary incontinence in 86%, pseudobulbar palsy in 52%)
   - Cognitive deficits in 48% (dementia 28%)
   - Migraines in up to 38%
   - Psychiatric disturbances in 30%
   - Seizures in 10%
   - Cognitive, gait problems can slowly worsen

- Suggestive diagnostic clues
   - Family history of strokes without risk factors
   - Family history of dementia
   - MRI often abnormal in presymptomatic patients; symmetric white matter, basal ganglia involvement with dramatic worsening over time
   - Normal CSF (rare cases of OCB positivity)

- Diagnosis involves gene testing, skin biopsy (osmiophilic deposition in vessel wall)

CVA, cerebrovascular accident; TIA, transient ischemic attack.

Eale's disease involves retinal perivasculitis and recurrent vitreous hemorrhages, with rare CNS vascular involvement.[158] This disorder affects young males (age 20–40 years). Patients present with sudden monocular vision loss, but ultimately both eyes are involved.

Hypertensive cerebrovascular disease, multiple cerebral emboli, and subcortical arteriosclerotic leukoencephalopathy (Binswanger disease) are vascular conditions which produce neurological problems and MRI abnormalities. MRI lesions are usually distinctly different from MS, and the clinical syndromes are more suggestive for stroke.

Periventricular leukomalacia affects preterm neonates. There are necrotic foci around the anterior and posterior ends of the lateral ventricles, as well as the centrum semiovale and the optic and acoustic radiations. MRI scans performed as an adult will detect these historic lesions as hyperintense on T2 and proton density scanning. The history of prematurity, as well as the presence of fixed neurological deficits dating to childhood, should be sufficient to recognize this entity.

Susac syndrome involves a microangiopathy of the retina, cochlea, and brain (Table 4.44).[159,160] In particular, the neuro-otologic features are most often misdiagnosed as MS. Treatment involves systemic immunosuppression.

Table 4.44 Susac syndrome.

- Retinocochleocerebral syndrome
- Noninflammatory vasculopathy with microinfarcts involving cochlea, retina, brain
- Mean age at onset 28 (range 18–59)
- Female predominance (>4 : 1)

Migraine can produce lesions on brain MRI. They are smaller and more peripheral than typical MS lesions. Vasculitis involving the CNS may be primary (primary CNS angiitis, or idiopathic granulomatous angiitis of the CNS), or secondary (systemic vasculitis, or vasculitis associated with collagen vascular disease or infection).[133] MRI lesions are often multifocal, bilateral, and involve both white and gray matter. Rarely they can be diffuse and symmetric, reminiscent of leukoencephalopathy.[161] Lesions may resolve with immunosuppressive therapy. Vasculitis can produce CSF pleocytosis and elevated protein concentration (often over 100 mg/dl). OCB may be present, but are unusual. Vasculitis patients often have headache and prominent mental status changes, as well as focal deficits.

Summary

It is important to be thorough in the initial assessment of a patient with suspected MS, to assure accurate diagnosis. Although the differential diagnosis is extensive, a thoughtful analysis will exclude other conditions. If the diagnosis remains uncertain, patients should be reassessed at a later timepoint since paraclinical test abnormalities increase over time. Accurate diagnosis remains the cornerstone to providing the best care for MS.

References

1. Allison RS, Millar JHD. Prevalence and familial incidence of disseminated sclerosis (a report to the Northern Ireland Hospitals Authority on the results of a three-year survey): prevalence of disseminated sclerosis in Northern Ireland. Ulster Med J 1954; 23:5–27.

2. Schumacher GA, Beebe G, Kibler RF, et al. Problems of experimental trials of therapy in multiple sclerosis. Report by the panel on the evaluation of experimental trials of therapy in multiple sclerosis. Ann NY Acad Sci 1965; 122:552–568.

3. Bauer J. IMAB-enquete concerning the diagnostic criteria for multiple sclerosis. In: Bauer HJ, Poser S, Ritter G, eds. Progress in multiple sclerosis research. Berlin: Springer; 1980: 555–563.

4. Poser CM, Paty DW, Scheinberg L, et al. New diagnostic criteria for multiple sclerosis: guidelines for research protocols. Ann Neurol 1983; 13:227–231.

5. Paty DW, Noseworthy JH, Ebers GC. Diagnosis of multiple sclerosis. In: Paty DW, Ebers GC, eds. Mutliple sclerosis. Philadelphia: FA Davis; 1998; 48–134.

6. McDonald WI, Compston A, Edan G, et al. Recommended diagnostic criteria for multiple sclerosis: guidelines from the International Panel on the diagnosis of multiple sclerosis. Ann Neurol 2001; 50:121–127.

7. Barkhof, Fillippi M, Miller DH, et al. Comparison of MR imaging criteria and first presentation to predict conversion to clinical definite multiple sclerosis. Brain 1997; 120:2059–2064.

8. Tintoré M, Rovifa A, Martinez M, et al. Isolated demyelinating syndromes: comparison of different MR imaging criteria to predict conversion to clinically definite multiple sclerosis. Am J Neuroradiol 2000; 21:702–706.

9. Paty DW, Li DK. Diagnosis of multiple sclerosis 1998: do we need new diagnostic criteria? In: Siva A, Kesselring J, Thompson AJ, eds. Frontiers in multiple sclerosis, vol 2. London: Martin Dunitz; 1999: 47–50.

10. Thompson AJ, Montalban X, Barkhof F, et al. Diagnostic criteria for primary progressive multiple sclerosis: a position paper. Ann Neurol 2000; 47:831–835.

11. Pöllmann W, Starck M, Albrecht H, König N. Late onset multiple sclerosis beyond the age of 60 years – a report of 15 cases. J Neurol Sci 2001; 187:S347.

12. Kira J-I, Kanai T, Nishimura Y, et al. Western versus Asian types of multiple sclerosis: immunogenetically and clinically distinct disorders. Ann Neurol 1996; 40:569–574.

13. Lublin FD, Reingold SC. Defining the clinical course of multiple sclerosis: results of an international survey. Neurology 1996; 46:907–911.

14. Andersson PB, Waubant E, Gee L, Goodkin DE. Multiple sclerosis that is progressive from the time of onset: clinical characteristics

and progression of disability. Arch Neurol 1999; 56:1138–1142.

15. Goodkin DE, Hertsgaard D, Rudick RA. Exacerbation rates and adherence to disease type in a prospectively followed-up population with multiple sclerosis. Implications for clinical trials. Arch Neurol 1989; 46:1107–1112.

16. Andersson M, Alvarez-Carmeno J, Bernardi G, et al. Cerebrospinal fluid in the diagnosis of multiple sclerosis: a consensus report. J Neurol Neurosurg Psychiatry 1994; 57:897–902.

17. Gronseth GS, Ashman EJ. Practice parameter: the usefulness of evoked potentials in identifying clinically silent lesions in patients with suspected multiple sclerosis (an evidence-based review). Report of the Quality Standards Subcommittee of the American Academy of Neurology. Neurology 2000; 54:1720–1725.

18. Flachenecker P, Reiners K, Krauser M, et al. Autonomic dysfunction in multiple sclerosis is related to disease activity and progression of disability. Mult Scler 2001; 7:327–334.

19. Merkelbach S, Dillmann U, Kölmel C, et al. Cardiovascular autonomic dysregulation and fatigue in multiple sclerosis. Mult Scler 2001; 7:320–326.

20. Yokota T, Matsunaga T, Okiyama R, et al. Sympathetic skin response in patients with multiple sclerosis compared with patients with spinal cord transection and normal controls. Brain 1991; 114:1381–1394.

21. Chabriat H, Vahedi K, Joutel A, et al. Cerebral autosomal dominant arteriopathy with subcortical infarcts and leukoencephalopathy (CADASIL). Neurologist 1997; 3:137–145.

22. Dichgans M, Mayer M, Uttner I, et al. The phenotypic spectrum of CADASIL: clinical findings in 102 cases. Ann Neurol 1998; 44:731–739.

23. Weinshenker BG, Lucchinetti CF. Acute leukoencephalopathics: differential diagnosis and investigation. Neurologist 1998; 4:148–166.

24. Haase CG, Faustmann PM, Diener HC. Acute disseminated encephalomyelitis (ADEM). Aktuelle Neurologie 1999; 26(2):68–71.

25. Ikeda Y, Sudoh A, Chiba S, Matsumoto H, Nakagawa T, Ohguro H. Detection of serum antibody against Arrestin from patients with acute disseminated encephalomyelitis. Tohoku J Exp Med 1999; 187:65–70.

26. Kesselring J, Miller DH, Robb SA, et al. Acute disseminated encephalomyelitis: MRI findings and the distinction from multiple sclerosis. Brain 1990; 113:291–302.

27. Tselis AC, Lisak RP. Acute disseminated encephalomyelitis. In: Antel J, Birnbaum G, Hartung H-P. (eds), Clinical Neuroimmunology. Massachusetts: Blackwell Science, 1998:16–147.

28. Saito H, Endo M, Takase S, Itahara K. Acute disseminated encephalomyelitis after influenza vaccination. Arch Neurol 1980; 37:564–566.

29. Alcock N, Hoffman H. Recurrent encephalomyelitis in childhood. Arch Dis Child 1962; 37:40–44.

30. Cohen O, Steiner-Birmanns B, Biran I, et al. Recurrence of acute disseminated encephalomyelitis at the previously affected brain site. Arch Neurol 2001; 58:797–801.

31. Khan S, Yaqub BA, Posner CM, et al. Multiphasic disseminated encephalomyelitis presenting as alternating hemiplegia. J Neurol Neurosurg Psychiatry 1995; 58:467–470.

32. Mizutani K, Atsuta J, Shibata T, et al. Consecutive cerebral MRI findings of acute relapsing disseminated encephalomyelitis. Acta Paediatr Jpn 1994; 36:709–712.

33. Johnson RT. Viral infections of the nervous system, 2nd edn. Philadelphia: Lippincott-Raven; 1998:181–210.

34. Atlas SW, Grossman RI, Goldberg HI, Hackney DB, Bilaniuk LT, Zimmerman RA. MR diagnosis of acute disseminated encephalomyelitis. J Comput Assist Tomogr 1986; 10:798–801.

35. Baum, PA, Barkovich J, Koch TK, Berg BO. Deep gray matter involvement in children with acute disseminated enchephalomyelitis. Am J Neurol 1994; 15:1275–1283.

36. Donovan M, Lenn N. Postinfectious encephalomyelitis with localized basal ganglia involvement. Pediatr Neurol 1962; 5:311–313.

37. Lukes S, Norman D. Computed tomography in acute disseminated encephalomyelitis. Ann Neurol 1983; 13:567–572.

38. Orrell RW, Shakir R, Lane RJM, et al. Distinguishing acute disseminated encephalomyelitis from multiple sclerosis. Br Med J 1996; 313:802–804.

39. Rust RS. Multiple sclerosis, acute disseminated encephalomyelitis, and related conditions. Semin Pediatr Neurol 2000; 2:66–90.

40. Schwartz S, Mohr A, Knauth M, et al. Acute disseminated encephalomyelitis. A follow-up study of 40 adult patients. Neurology 2001; 56:1313–1318.

41. Rust RS, Dodson W, Prensky A, et al. Classification and outcome of acute disseminated encephalomyelitis. Ann Neurol 1997; 42:491.

42. Dale RC, DeSousa C, Chong WK, et al. Acute disseminated encephalomyelitis, multiple disseminated encephalomyelitis and MS in children. Brain 2000; 123:2407–2422.

43. Abramsky O, Teitelbaum D, Arnon R. Effect of a synthetic polypeptide (cop-1) on patients with multiple sclerosis and with acute disseminated encephalomyelitis. J Neurol Sci 1977; 31:433–438.

44. Hahn JS, Siegler DJ, Enzmann D. Intravenous gammaglobulin therapy in recurrent acute disseminated encephalomyelitis. Neurology 1996; 46:1173–1174.

45. Kleiman M, Brunquell P. Acute disseminated encephalomyelitis: response to intravenous immunoglobulin? J Child Neurol 1995; 10:481–483.

46. Salazar AM, Engel WK, Levy HB. Poly ICLC in the treatment of postinfectious demyelinating encephalomyelitis. Arch Neurol 1981; 38:382–383.

47. Hurst E. Acute haemorrhagic leucoencephalitis: a previous undefined entity. Med J Aust 1941; 2:1–6.

48. Hart M, Earle K. Haemorrhagic and perivenous encephalitis: a clinical-pathological review of 38 cases. J Neurol Neurosurg Psychiatry 1975; 38:585–591.

49. O'Riordan JI, Thompson AJ, Kingsley DPE, et al. The prognostic value of brain MRI in clinically isolated syndromes of the CNS. A 10-year follow-up. Brain 1998; 121:495–503.

50. Sailer M, O'Riordan JI, Thomas AJ, et al. Quantitative MRI in patients with clinically isolated syndromes suggestive of demyelination. Neurology 1999; 52:599–606.

51. Optic Neuritis Study Group. The 5-year risk of MS after optic neuritis. Experience of the optic neuritis treatment trial. Neurology 1997; 49:1404–1413.

52. Lucchinetti C, Kiers L, O'Duffy A, et al. Risk factors for developing multiple sclerosis after childhood optic neuritis. Neurology 1997; 49:1413–1418.

53. Devic E. Myelite subaigue compliquee de neurite optique. Bull Med 1894; 5:18–30.

54. Silber MH, Willcox PA, Bowen RM, Unger A. Neuromyelitis optica (Devic's syndrome) and pulmonary tuberculosis. Neurology 1990; 40:934–938.

55. Whitham RH, Brey RL. Neuromyelitis optica: two new cases and review of the literature. J Clin Neurol-ophthalmol 1985; 5:263–269.

56. Hogancamp W, Weinshenker B. The spectrum of Devic's syndrome. Neurology 1996; 46(S):254 [abstract].

57. Wingerchuck DM, Hogancamp WF, O'Brien PC, Weinshenker BG. The clinical course of neuromyelitis optica (Devic's syndrome) Neurology 1999; 53:1107–1114.

58. Leonardi A, Arata L, Farinelli M, et al. Cerebrospinal fluid and neuropathological study in Devic's syndrome. Evidence of intrathecal immune activation. J Neurol Sci 1987; 82:281–290.

59. Mandler R, Davis LE, Jeffery DR, Kornfeld M. Devic's neuromyelitis optica: a clinicopathological study of 8 patients. Ann Neurol 1993; 34:162–168.

60. Mandler RN, Ahmed W, Agius M, et al. Devic's neuromyelitis optica. Pathogenic characteristics and favorable response to immunotherapy in six acute patients. Mult Scler 1997; 3:407 [abstract].

61. O'Riordan JI, Gallagher HL, Thomson AJ, et al. Clinical, CSF, and MRI findings in Devic's neuromyelitis optica. J Neurol Neurosurg Psychiatry 1996; 60:382–387.

62. Piccolo G, Franciotta DM, Camana C, et al. Devic's neuromyelitis optica: long-term follow-up and serial CSF finding in two cases. J Neurol 1990; 237:262–264.

63. Jeffery AR, Buncic JR. Pediatric Devic's neuromyelitis optica. J Pediatr Ophthalmol Strabismus 1996; 33(s):223–229.

64. Arnold TW, Myers GJ. Neuromyelitis optica (Devic's syndrome) in a 12-year-old male with complete recovery following steroids. Pediatr Neurol 1987; 3:313–315.

65. Mandler RN, Ahmed W, Dencoff JE. Devic's neuromyelitis optica: a progressive study of seven patients treated with prednisone and azathioprine. Neurology 1998; 51:1219–1220.

66. Rensel MR, Weinstock-Guttman B, Rudick R. Devic's disease: diagnostic and therapeutic challenge. Mult Scler 1997; 3(s):408.

67. Aguilera AJ, Carlow TJ, Smith KJ, Simon TL. Lymphocytaplasmapheresis in Devic's syndrome. Transfusion 1985; 25:54–56.

68. Haase CG, Schmidt S. Detection of brain-specific autoantibodies to myelin oligodendrocyte glycoprotein, S100beta and myelin basic protein in patients with Devic's neuromyelitis optica. Neurosci Lett 2001; 307:131–133.

69. Bitsch A, Wegener C, da Costa C, et al. Lesion development in Marburg's type of acute multiple sclerosis: from inflammation to demyelination. Mult Scler 1999; 5:138–146.

70. Giubilei F, Sarrantonio A, Tisei P, et al. Four year follow-up of a case of acute multiple sclerosis of the Marburg type. Ital J Neurol Sci 1997; 18:163–166.

71. Johnson MD, Lavin P. Whetsell WO Jr. Fulminant monophasic multiple sclerosis, Marburg's

type. J Neurol Neurosurg Psychiatry 1990; 53:918–921.

72. Marburg O. Die Sogenannte "akute multiple sklerose" (encephalomyelitis periacialis scleroticans). J Psychict Neurol 1906; 27:211–312.

73. Mendez MF, Pogacar S. Malignant monophasic mulltiple sclerosis or "Marburg's disease". Neurology 1998; 38:1153–1155.

74. Wood DD, Bibao JM, O'Connors P, Moscarello MA. Acute multiple sclerosis (Marburg type) is associated with developmentally immature myelin basic protein. Ann Neurol 1996; 40:18–24.

75. Ernst T, Chang L, Walot I, Huff K. Physiologic MRI of a tumefactive multiple sclerosis lesion. Neurology 1998; 51:1486–1488.

76. Dagher AP, Smirniotopoulos J. Tumefactive demyelinating lesions. Neuroradiology 1996; 38:560–565.

77. Giang DW, Poduri KR, Eskin TA, et al. Multiple sclerosis masquerading as a mass lesion. Neuroradiology 1992; 34:150–154.

78. Hunter S, Ballinger W, Rubin J. Multiple sclerosis mimicking primary brain tumor. Arch Pathol Lab Med 1987; 111:464–468.

79. Mastrostefano R, Occhipinti E, Bigotti G, Pompili A. Multiple sclerosis plaque simulating cerebral tumor: case report and review of the literature. Neurosurgery 1987; 21:244–246.

80. Rieth K, Di Chiro G, Cromwell L. Primary demyelinating disease simulating glioma of the corpus collosum: report of three cases. Neurosurgery 1981; 55:620–624.

81. Kepes JJ. Large focal tumor-like demyelinating lesions of the brain: intermediate entity between multiple sclerosis and acute disseminated encephalomyelitis? A study of 31 patients. Ann Neurol 1993; 33:18–27.

82. Balo J. Encephalitis periaxialis concentrica. Arch Neurol Psychiatry 1928; 19:242–264.

83. Castaigne P, Escourolle R, Chain F, et al. Balo's concentric sclerosis. Rev Neurol (Paris) 1984; 140:479–487.

84. Currie S, Roberts AH, Urich H. The nosological position of concentric lacunar leukoencephalopathy. J Neurol Neurosurg Psychiatry 1970; 33:131–137.

85. Garbern J, Spence AM, Alvord EC Jr. Balo's concentric demyelination diagnosed premortem. Neurology 1986; 36:1610–1614.

86. Gharagozloo A, Poe L, Collins G. Antemortem diagnosis of Balo concentric sclerosis: correlative neuroimaging and pathological features. Radiology 1994; 191:817–819.

87. Itoyama Y, Tateishi J, Kuroiwa Y. Atypical multiple sclerosis with concentric or lamellar demyelination lesions: two Japanese patients studied post mortem. Ann Neurol 1985; 17:481–487.

88. Moore GRW, Neumann PE, Suzuki K, et al. Balo's concentric sclerosis: new observations on lesion development. Ann Neurol 1985; 17:604–611.

89. Murakami Y, Matsuishi T, Shimizu T, et al. Balo's concentric sclerosis in a 4-year old Japanese infant. Brain Devel 1998; 20:250–252.

90. Nandini M, Gourie-Devi M, Shankar SK, et al. Balo's concentric sclerosis diagnosed intravitum on brain biopsy. Clin Neurol Neurosurg 1993; 95:303–309.

91. Yao D, Webster HD, Hudson LD, Brenner M, et al. Concentric sclerosis (Balo): morphometric and in situ hybridization study of lesions in six patients. Ann Neurol 1994; 5:18–30.

92. Lucchinetti C, Brück W, Parisi J, et al. Heterogeneity of multiple sclerosis lesions: implications for

the pathogenesis of demyelination. Ann Neurol 2000; 47:707–717.

93. Chen C, Ro LS, Chang CN, Ho YS, Lu CS. Serial MRI studies in pathologically verified Balo's concentric sclerosis. J Comput Assist Tomogr 1996; 20:732–735.

94. Hanemann CO, Kleinschmidt A, Reifenberger G, et al. Balo's concentric sclerosis followed by MRI and positron emission tomography. Neuroradiology 1993; 35:578–580.

95. Korte J, Born EP, Vos LD, et al. Balo's concentric sclerosis: MR diagnosis. Am J Neuroradiol 1994; 15:1284–1288.

96. Louboutin J, Elie B. Treatment of Balo's concentric sclerosis with immunosuppressant drugs followed by multimodality evoked potentials and MRI. Muscle Nerve 1995; 18:1478–1480.

97. Sekijima Y, Tokuda T, Hashimoto T, et al. Serial magnetic resonance imaging (MRI) study of a patient with Balo's concentric sclerosis treated with immunadsorption plasmapheresis. Mult Scler 1997; 2:291–294.

98. Spiegel M, Kruger H, Hoffmann E, Kappos L. MRI study of Balo's concentric sclerosis before and after immunosuppressant therapy. J Neurol 1989; 236:487–488.

99. Canavan NM. Schilder's encephalitis periaxialis diffusa. Report of a case in a child aged sixteen and one half months. Arch Neurol 1931; 25:229–308.

100. Eblen F, Poremba M, Grodd W, Opitz H, Roggendorf W, Dichgans J. Myelinoclastic diffuse sclerosis (Schilder's disease): cliniconeuroradiologic correlations. Neurology 1991; 41:589–591.

101. Mehler MF, Rabinowich L. Inflammatory myelinoclastic diffuse sclerosis. Ann Neurol 1988; 23:413–415.

102. Poser CM, Goutieres F, Carpentier MA, Aicardi J. Schilder's myelinoclastic diffuse sclerosis. Pediatrics 1986; 77:107–112.

103. Schilder P. Zur Frage derencephalitis periaxialis diffusa. Z Gesamte Neurol Psychiat 1913; 15:359–376.

104. Pretorius M-L, Looke DB, Ravenscroft A, Schoeman JF. Demyelinating disease of Schilder type in three young South African children: dramatic response to corticosteriods. J Child Neurol 1998; 13:197–201.

105. Galaburda AM, Waxman SG, Kemper TL, Jones HR. Progressive multifocal neurological deficit with disseminated subpial demyelination. J Neuropathol Exp Neurol 1976; 35:481–494.

106. Neumann PE, Mehler MF, Horoupian DS, Merriam AE. Atypical psychosis with disseminated subpial demyelination. Arch Neurol 1988; 45:634–636.

107. Herndon RM, Brooks B. Misdiagnosis of multiple sclerosis. Semin Neurol 1985; 5:94–98.

108. Rudick RA, Schiffer RB, Schwetz M, Herndon RM. Multiple sclerosis: the problem of incorrect diagnosis. Arch Neurol 1986; 43:578–583.

109. Pullicino P, Ostrow PT, Kwen PL. Cerebral white matter disease: imaging, clinical, and pathological aspects. Neurologist 1996; 2:288–301.

110. Triulzi F, Scotti G. Differential diagnosis of multiple sclerosis: contribution of magnetic resonance techniques. J Neurol Neurosurg Psychiatry 1998; 64:S6–S14.

111. Natowicz MR, Bejjani B. Genetic disorders that masquerade as multiple sclerosis. Am J Med Genet 1994; 49:149–169.

112. Mitsias P, Levine SR. Cerebrovascular complications of Fabry's

disease. Ann Neurol 1996; 40:8–17.

113. Klemm E, Conzelmann E. Adult-onset metachromatic leucodystrophy presenting without psychiatric symptoms. J Neurol 1989; 236:427–429.

114. DiMauro S, DeVivo DC. Genetic heterogeneity in Leigh syndrome. Ann Neurol 1996; 40:5–7.

115. Baumgartner MR, Poll-The BT, Verhoeven NM, et al. Clinical approach to inherited peroxisomal disorders: a series of 27 patients. Ann Neurol 1998; 44:720–730.

116. Moser HW, Raymond GV. Genetic peroxisomal disorders: why, when, and how to test. Ann Neurol 1998; 44:713–714.

117. Brewer GJ. Recognition, diagnosis, and management of Wilson's disease. Proc Soc Exp Biol Med. 2000; 223:39–46.

118. Schiefermeier M, Kollegger H, Madl C, et al. The impact of apolipoprotein E genotypes on age at onset of symptoms and phenotypic expression in Wilson's disease. Brain 2000; 123:585–590.

119. Enbom M. Human herpesvirus 6 in the pathogenesis of multiple sclerosis. APMIS 2001; 109: 401–411.

120. Knox KK, Brewer JH, Henry JM, Harrington DJ, Carrigan DR. Human herpesvirus 6 and multiple sclerosis: systemic active infections in patients with early disease. Clin Infect Dis. 2000; 31:894–903.

121. Manji H, Miller RF. Progressive multifocal leucoencephalopathy: progress in the AIDS era. J Neurol Neurosurg Psychiatry. 2000; 69:569–571.

122. Berger JR, Sheremata WA, Resnick L, et al. Multiple sclerosis-like illness occurring with human immunodeficiency virus infection. Neurology 1989; 39:324–329.

123. Berger JR, Tornatore C, Major EO, et al. Relapsing and remitting human immunodeficiency virus-associated leukoencephalomyelopathy. Ann Neurol 1992; 31:34–38.

124. Gray F, Chimelli L, Mohr M, et al. Fulminating multiple sclerosis-like leukoencephalopathy revealing human immunodeficiency virus infection. Neurology 1991; 41:105–109.

125. Nagai M, Jacobson S. Immunopathogenesis of human T cell lymphotropic virus type I-associated myelopathy. Curr Opin Neurol 2001; 14:381–386.

126. Yucesan C. Sriram S. *Chlamydia pneumoniae* infection of the central nervous system. Curr Opin Neurol 2001; 14:355–359.

127. Bussone G, La Mantia L, Grazzi L, et al. Neurobrucellosis mimicking multiple sclerosis: a case report. Eur Neurol 1989; 29:238–240.

128. Coyle PK, Schutzer SE. Neurologic aspects of Lyme disease. Med Clin N Am 2002; 86:1–24.

129. Coban O, Bahar S, Akman-Demir G, et al. Misled assembly of MRI findings: is it possible to differentiate neuro-Behçet's disease from other CNS disease? Neuroradiology 1999; 41:255–260.

130. Kansu T. Neuro-Behçet's disease. Neurologist 1998; 4:31–39.

131. Kocer N, Islak C, Siva A, et al. CNS involvement in neuro-Behçet syndrome: a MR study. Am J Neuroradiol 1999; 20:1015–1024.

132. Serdaroglu P. Behçet's disease and the nervous system. J Neurol 1998; 245:197–205.

133. Kira J, Goto I. Recurrent opticomyelitis associated with anti-DNA antibody. J Neurol Neurosurg Psychiatry 1994; 57:1124–1125.

134. Moore PM, Richardson B. Neurology of the vasculitides and connective tissue diseases. J Neurol Neurosurg Psychiatry 1998; 65:10–22.

135. De Seze J, Devos D, Castelnovo G, et al. The prevalence of Sjögren syndrome in patients with primary progressive multiple sclerosis. Neurology 2001; 57:1359–1363.

136. Scott TF. Neurosarcoidosis: progress and clinical aspects. Neurology. 1993; 43:8–12.

137. Zajicek JP, Scolding NJ, Foster O, et al. Central nervous system sarcoidosis – diagnosis and management. Q J Med 1999; 92:103–117.

138. Chatterjee A, Yapundich R, Palmer CA, et al. Leukoencephalopathy associated with cobalamin deficiency. Neurology 1996; 46:824–832.

139. Aparicio JM, Belanger-Quintana A, Suarez L, et al. Ataxia with isolated vitamin E deficiency: case report and review of the literature. J Pediatr Gastroenterol Nutr 2001; 33:206–210.

140. Gabsi S, Gouider-Khouja N, Belal S, et al. Effect of vitamin E supplementation in patients with ataxia with vitamin E deficiency. Eur J Neurol 2001; 8:477–481.

141. Fukuda K, Straus SE, Hickie I, Sharpe MC, Dobbins JG, Komaroff A. The chronic fatigue syndrome: a comprehensive approach to its definition and study. International Chronic Fatigue Syndrome Study Group. Ann Intern Med 1994; 121:953–959.

142. Natelson BH. Chronic fatigue syndrome. JAMA 2001; 285:2557–2559.

143. Brazis PW, Lee AG. Optic disk edema with a macular star. Mayo Clin Proc 1996; 71:1162–1166.

144. Smith ME, Katz DA, Harris JO, et al. Systemic histiocytosis presenting as multiple sclerosis. Ann Neurol 1993; 33:549–554.

145. Deen HG, Nelson KD, Gonzales GR. Spinal dural arteriovenous fistula causing progressive myelopathy: clinical and imaging considerations. Mayo Clin Proc 1994; 69:83–84.

146. Flippo T, Holder W Jr. Neurologic degeneration associated with nitrous oxide anesthesia in patients with vitamin B_{12} deficiency. Arch Surg 1993; 39:659–667.

147. Small SL, Fukui MB, Bramblett GT, Eidelman BH. Immunosuppression-induced leukoencephalopathy from tacrolimus (FK506). Ann Neurol 1996; 40:575–580.

148. Arbiser JL, Kraeft SK, van Leeuwen R, et al. Clioquinol-zinc chelate: a candidate causative agent of subacute myelo-optic neuropathy. Mol Med 1998; 4:665–670.

149. Tateishi J. Subacute myelo-optico-neuropathy: clioquinol intoxication in humans and animals. Neuropathology 2000; 20:S20–S24.

150. Cuadro MJ, Khamashta MS, Ballesteros A, et al. Can neurologic manifestations of Hughes (Antiphospolipid) Syndrome be distinguished from MS? Medicine 2000; 79:57–68.

151. Levine S, Brey R. Neurological aspects of antiphospholipid antibody syndrome. Lupus 1996; 5:346–353.

152. Chabriat H, Levy C, Taillia H, et al. Patterns of MRI lesions in CADASIL. Neurology 1998; 51:452–457.

153. Coulthard A, Blank SC, Bushby K, et al. Distribution of clinical MRI abnormalities in patients with symptomatic and subclinical CADASIL. Br J Radiol 2000; 73:256–265.

154. Ceroni M, Bloni TE, Tonietti S, et al. Migraine with aura and white

matter abnormalities: notch 3 mutation. Neurology 2000; 54:1869–1871.

155. Desmond DW, Moroney JT, Lynch T, et al. CADASIL in a North American family. Clinical, pathological, and radiologic findings. Neurology 1998; 51:844–849.

156. Filley CM, Thompson LL, Sze C-I, et al. White matter dementia in CADASIL. J Neurol Sci 1999; 163:163–167.

157. Yousry TA, Selos K, Mayer H, et al. Characteristic MRI lesion pattern and correlation of T1 and T2 lesion white matter with neurologic and neurophysiologic findings in CADASIL. Am J Neuroradiol 1999; 20:91–100.

158. Gordon MF, Coyle PK, Golub B. Eale's disease presenting as stroke in the young adult. Ann Neurol 1988; 24: 264–266.

159. Papo T, Biousse V, Lehoang P, et al. Susac syndrome. Medicine 1998; 77:3–11.

160. Susac JO. Susac's syndrome: the triad of microangiopathy of the brain and retina with hearing loss in young women. Neurology 1994; 44:591–593.

161. Finelli PF, Onyiuke HC, Uphoff DF. Idiopathic granulomatous angiitis of the NCS manifesting as diffuse white matter disease. Neurology 1997; 49:1696–1699.

5
Clinical features

Initial manifestations

The clinical manifestations of MS are extremely protean. Indeed, virtually any neurological symptom or sign has been described. However, certain features are characteristic and often appear early in the course of the disease, whereas other clinical problems tend to occur later. Probably most common among the initial presentations of the disease are somatosensory symptoms.[1-3] Patients most often complain of "numbness" by which they usually mean a subjectively positive sensation, rather than diminished or absent sensation. These positive symptoms may include tingling, a feeling as if the body part is "asleep," tightness, burning, a feeling as if "procaine (Novacaine) is wearing off," or a sensation as if a garment such as a glove, a sock, or a girdle is present on the relevant body part. The abnormal sensation often occurs in a band-like fashion around the abdomen or a limb, and sometimes only a patch of abnormal sensation is reported. Typically these complaints are unaccompanied by objective signs on the neurological examination. This fact, coupled with the peculiar distributions of the symptoms, which often do not correspond to recognized dermatomal, peripheral nerve, or homuncular patterns, often leads to a failure of the physician to realize the clinical importance of the complaints. Not uncommonly, patients are told "it's your nerves," a truth to be sure, but not reflecting the clinician's actual understanding of the situation.

Motor symptoms, most often in one or both lower extremities, represent another category of commonly seen initial manifestations. More detailed discussion will be provided below.

The third very common initial presentation of MS is optic neuritis. With this condition, patients usually complain of unilateral dimming of vision. This may only be realized when the patient covers one eye, for example when a woman is applying makeup. The visual impairment is often accompanied by photophobia and pain aggravated by eye movement. Examination reveals diminished visual acuity which varies greatly in severity, from mere decrease in color saturation to complete monocular blindness, though the latter is uncommon. Formal visual field examination most typically reveals a central or paracentral scotoma (Figure 5.1).

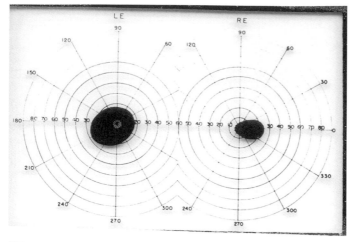

(A)

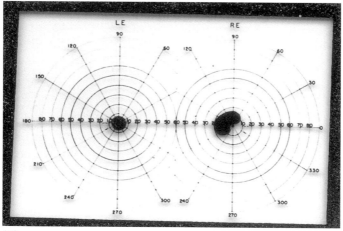

(B)

Figure 5.1
Scotomas: (A) left paracentral scotoma, right cecocentral scotoma; (B) left central scotoma, right paracentral scotoma (courtesy of Dr. Arthur Wolintz).

Fundoscopy may show a swollen optic nerve head with hemorrhages or exudates (papillitis), (Figure 5.2) but more often a normal optic disc (retrobulbar neuritis) is found. In fact, in an isolated case of optic neuritis, the finding of papillitis conveys a lower risk of subsequent development of clinically definite MS which may otherwise occur in 30–80% of cases, dependent, at least in part, on the duration of follow-up. Fortunately, good recovery of vision is usual, even when the initial visual loss is quite severe.

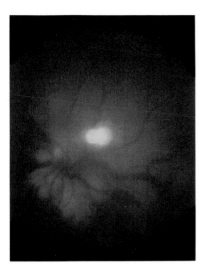

Figure 5.2
Fundus photograph showing markedly swollen optic nerve head of papillitis. Most cases of acute optic neuritis in MS show relatively normal disks as the lesions are typically retrobulbar (courtesy of Dr. Arthur Wolintz).

Course and prognosis

The course of MS is extremely variable and offering reliable prognosis for an individual patient, especially early in the illness, is difficult, if not impossible. Because physicians, including MS specialists, were using different terms to describe patients, a few years ago Lublin and Reingold sought consensus among many MS experts. Consensus definitions were necessitated by the lack of reliable biological, immunological, or radiological markers that distinguish among the different disease courses. The authors defined four temporal patterns of the disease (Figure 5.3), providing a descriptive terminology that has subsequently been widely used (Table 4.8).[4]

The vast majority of patients (80–85%) start with a pattern marked by exacerbations – also referred to as attacks or relapses – and remissions. An exacerbation is usually conventionally defined as the development of new symptoms lasting at least 24 hours and separated from a previous attack by at least a month (Table 5.1). This form of the disease is described as relapsing-remitting MS (RRMS). The individual attacks may be followed by either complete or partial recovery, with the critical feature the fact that the patient remains clinically stable until the next discrete exacerbation. Thus, it is possible for a patient's course to be described as relapsing-remitting even if cumulative disability has occurred, provided that the worsening developed only as a result of clearly discernible relapses.

Clinical Patterns of MS

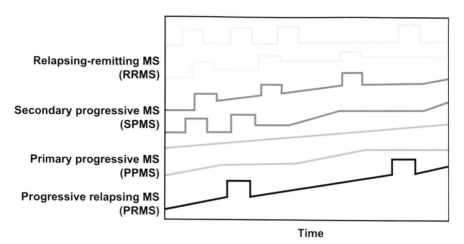

Relapsing-remitting MS
(RRMS)

Secondary progressive MS
(SPMS)

Primary progressive MS
(PPMS)

Progressive relapsing MS
(PRMS)

Time

Figure 5.3
MS has been subdivided into four types by consensus of specialists. Most patients begin with relapsing-remitting disease. Many of these change to secondary progressive disease during which they worsen between attacks or in their absence. About 10-15% of patients begin with primary progressive disease, whereas the progressive-relapsing form is very uncommon.

Table 5.1 Characteristic MS clinical relapses.

- Motor abnormalities (weakness, spasticity)
- Sensory disturbances (numbness, paresthesias, pain, Lhermitte sign)
- Cerebellar abnormalities (incoordination, imbalance, tremor)
- Vision disturbances (monocular decrease in vision and color perception, with eye pain)
- Brainstem abnormalities (diplopia, trigeminal neuralgia, internuclear ophthalmoplegia)
- Bladder difficulties (urgency, frequency, overflow leakage, incontinence, inability to void)
- Bowel difficulties (constipation; rarely diarrhea, fecal incontinence)
- Sexual dysfunction
- Cognitive difficulty

A much smaller group of patients, approximately 10–15%, never experience acute attacks, instead developing progressive disability from the onset. Plateaus in the clinical status, but no significant improvement, may occur. This form of the disease, termed primary progressive MS (PPMS), may differ biologically from other forms of the illness. Patients with PPMS are frequently older (over the age of 40) when the disease becomes evident, have a more even gender distribution (1 : 1 rather than the 3 : 2 or 2 : 1

female to male ratio reported for RRMS), and tend to manifest progressive spastic paraparesis. Cranial MRI shows relatively fewer abnormalities and recent reports suggest some pathological differences.

A very small number of patients (probably fewer than 5%) have a course termed progressive-relapsing MS. These individuals begin worsening gradually, as if they will have PPMS, but subsequently start to experience discrete attacks.

Unfortunately, most patients (probably 50–60%) with RRMS change over time to a pattern in which their clinical condition gradually worsens. This temporal profile is then termed secondary progressive MS (SPMS). Some patients with SPMS no longer experience any discernible exacerbations. Others do continue to experience attacks, but the hallmark of SPMS is detectable worsening either between or in the absence of relapses. That is, the stable clinical baseline that exists between attacks even in a deteriorating RRMS patient is lacking.

In a typical case of MS, the initial attack resolves completely, or nearly so, with the patient remaining entirely well until the next discrete exacerbation. This generally occurs within a few years; in one series 25% relapsed within one year and 50% within three years.[2] However, it is not rare to encounter patients who have had a latent period of many years between their first and second episodes. This is particularly true if one takes a very careful history seeking evidence for early symptoms, most often sensory, for which the patient may not even have sought medical attention. The average attack rate has varied from 0.1 to 0.85 annually in several series.[2] Clinical trials, selecting patients who have experienced recently active disease, have reported attack rates in placebo-treated patients ranging from 0.87 to 1.3 annually. [5-7] In most such studies, however, diminishing attack rates have occurred over the course of the trials.

The usual exacerbation develops over hours to days, although at times the onset may be so abrupt as to suggest the onset of a stroke. Conversely, attacks may occasionally develop in a more indolent fashion. Symptoms tend to remit within a week to a few months. In one series, when patients were seen within 2 months, 85% of relapses remitted completely. However, among patients not seen until 3 months, the rate fell to 30% and to only 10% for those seen at 6 months.[3] Gadolinium enhancement on MRI, currently regarded as the best imaging marker of recent disease activity, tends to persist for about 4–6 weeks, providing support for the clinical observations about the duration of attacks.

For those patients with progressing disease, deterioration tends to continue, albeit usually at a relatively slow rate. In a large natural history study, Weinshenker et al noted that 50% of patients required at least unilateral assistance to walk by 15 years after the onset of symptoms.[8] The Kurtzke Expanded Disability Status Scale (EDSS) has been widely used to rate the neurological status of MS patients (Figure 5.4). It is a 10 point scale, divided into half steps.[9,10] In general, patients scoring ≤3.5 have mini-

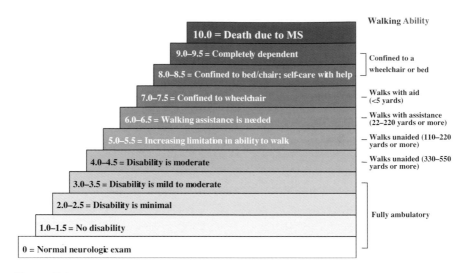

Figure 5.4
The Kurtzke Expanded Disability Status Scale (EDSS) is the most widely used measure of disability in MS. (Adapted from Kurtzke JF. Rating neurologic impairment in multiple sclerosis: an expanded disability status scale {EDSS}. Neurology 1983; 33: 144–142)

mal disability, at 6.0 patients require unilateral assistance to walk, 6.5 bilateral assistance, and at 7.0 are essentially wheelchair dependent. In one series, scoring patients with the EDSS, those who were ambulatory when initially evaluated worsened by 1.0–1.5 steps, on average, over the next 5 years. Those who required assistance to walk or were wheelchair dependent on entry into the study worsened by 0.3–0.7 steps over that period of observation. In one clinical trial, however, in which patients were selected because they appeared to be following a progressive course, approximately 20% demonstrated little or no worsening over the next 12 months.[11]

Multiple sclerosis can also be categorized by outcome. At the extremes, MS can be characterized as either benign or malignant, with most cases falling along a spectrum between these poles.

Benign MS has been defined as disease that allows patients to remain fully functional in all neurological systems 15 years after disease onset. Although this form may comprise 10–15% of patients, diagnosis, and thus prognosis, is difficult, and by definition requires a long passage of time. Even after many years, relapses and/or progression can occur, sometimes as late as 25 or more years later.

Malignant MS, on the other hand, is defined as disease with a rapid, progressive course, leading to significant disability in multiple neurological systems or death in a relatively short time after disease onset. This is, fortunately, quite rare.

In most studies, MS does not have a major impact on life expectancy. Wynn et al found a 74% survival rate at 25 years, compared with an expected rate of 86%.[12] In another series, Kurtzke et al similarly found 75% of normal survival in that period.[13]

The disease, overall, worsens over the years in more than 80% of patients. Studies have shown only 11–34% of patients able to work within 15 years of onset. However, at times MS follows an extremely benign course, with 10–20% of patients remaining with no significant neurological disability 25 or more years after the initial manifestations.

It must be emphasized that these data derive from natural history studies prior to the availability of the immunomodulatory drugs, which were introduced to the marketplace beginning in 1993. The hope, of course, is that these agents which reduced relapse rates by approximately 30% during the 2- to 3-year periods of the clinical trials, will ultimately convert more patients to benign forms of the disease with much less disability developing over time. Longer term follow-up of patients will be necessary to address this issue.

Although the long term behavior of groups of MS patients is understood, it is extremely difficult to offer an accurate prognosis to an individual, especially early in the course of the disease. The best predictor is how one is doing after 5 years or, still better, after 10 years, as the disease then tends to follow a similar pattern. For the patient with early disease, however, one can offer information based only on features that augur relatively weakly for a more or less favorable course. Indicators of a less severe course include early age of onset, female sex, optic neuritis or sensory symptoms as the presenting episode, acute onset of symptoms, little residual disability after each exacerbation, and long period of stability between the initial exacerbations (Table 5.2). By con-

Table 5.2 Favorable prognostic indicators in MS.

- Early age of onset
- Female sex
- Optic neuritis as presenting symptom
- Sensory symptoms as presenting episode
- Acute onset of symptoms
- Little residual disability after each exacerbation
- Long interexacerbation period

Table 5.3 Unfavorable prognostic indicators in MS.

- Later age of onset
- Progressive course from onset
- Male sex
- Frequent exacerbations
- Poor recovery from exacerbations
- Involvement of cerebellar and/or motor functions

trast, less favorable prognostic indicators include later age of onset, progressive course from onset, male sex, frequent exacerbations, poor recovery from exacerbations, and involvement of cerebellar and/or motor functions early in the course (Table 5.3).

Few aggravating factors have been convincingly demonstrated for MS. Viral infections seem to be the most clearly established precipitant of exacerbations, perhaps by stimulating interferon gamma, which may, in turn, cause increased antigen presentation and thereby trigger the attack. Panitch et al reported a clinical trial in which investigators hoped that interferon gamma would have a therapeutic effect. Rather, its administration promptly resulted in exacerbations in 7 of 18 patients treated within the month of treatment, an astonishingly high rate.[14]

Over the years, many claims have been made that both physical and psychological stress could precipitate worsening of MS. However, a detailed controlled study showed no significant association between any form of trauma and an increased frequency of attacks.[15] Similarly, reports that surgery or anesthesia could trigger deterioration have been unsubstantiated. A recently published review by a committee of the American Academy of Neurology, after extensive consideration of the evidence, found no relationship between physical trauma and MS exacerbation.[16] This same group, however, was less decisive about the possible relationship of psychological stress and MS.[16]

The assessment of the possible role of psychological stress in MS has been beset by many methodological problems. These include difficulties in measuring stress (inadequacies of psychological tests); recall bias; and the use of small or biased samples. Some recent studies, including observations of increased disease activity on cranial MRI have suggested that psychological factors may worsen MS. This is certainly conceivable in view of the fact that investigations in laboratory animals have shown changes in the immune system as a result of psychological stress. By contrast, however, during the presumably stressful period of SCUD missile attacks on Israel during the Gulf war, the exacerbation rate actually declined.[17]

Transient worsening of neurological symptoms in MS may occur in a number of circumstances. Best documented is worsening associated with elevations in body temperature. Thus, pseudoexacerbations may develop in the setting of fever, with the rapid resolution of the neurological deterioration when the elevated temperature is lowered. The observation that even a slight rise in temperature can produce new symptoms or worsening of existing ones was the basis for the hot bath test, a diagnostic tool rarely, if ever, used today. In this test, individuals suspected of MS, but perhaps with clinical findings in only one anatomical area, were placed in a bath with the water warm enough to raise body temperature a degree or so. The patient was then observed to see if additional neurological signs would develop. Provocation of neurological worsening, most typically blurring of vision, has also been reported with even moderate exercise. Known as Uhthoff's phenomenon, this, too, most likely results from a slight elevation in core body temperature which presumably causes increased neurological dysfunction as a result of the development of conduction block in partially demyelinated axons.

Pregnancy

Although early authors suggested that pregnancy might have an adverse effect on the course of MS, a number of more modern investigations re-examined this question both retrospectively and prospectively (Table 5.4).[18-23] Most, but not all, recent reports have indicated that patients tend to have fewer exacerbations during the pregnancy, but experience an increased attack rate in the postpartum period. Confavreux et al conducted the largest prospective study, following 254 women with MS in 12 European countries through 269 pregnancies.[22] Relapse rate reduction occurred throughout pregnancy, but most convincingly in the third trimester when the attack rate decreased to 0.2 ± 1.0 compared with 0.7 ± 0.9 during the year preceding the pregnancy ($P < 0.001$). However, the rate then rose significantly above that of the pre-pregnancy year during the first 3 months postpartum to 1.2 ± 2.0 before returning to baseline. Breast-feeding did not seem to have an impact on the relapse rate. Possible factors related to the increased postpartum attack frequency may be changes in immunological status after pregnancy, hormonal changes, or the stress and fatigue associated with caring for a newborn infant. Current evidence does not indicate any long-term negative influence of pregnancy on the course of MS, with some recent reports, in fact, suggesting a better prognosis.[23,24]

Table 5.4 Pregnancy issues

- Relapse rate
  - During pregnancy
  - During post-partum period

- Genetics

- Use of medications
  - During pregnancy
  - During breastfeeding

- Child-rearing

Specific clinical manifestations

Motor

Motor manifestations are among the more common early symptoms of MS, occurring with the initial attack in 32–41% of patients.[2] However, ultimately a substantial majority of patients (62% in one series) experience corticospinal[1,3] tract involvement. Patients frequently experience weakness, but may also complain of "heaviness," "stiffness," or even pain in an extremity. The motor symptoms typically begin in the lower extremities, often in one leg, but sometimes bilaterally. Occasionally an arm may be involved initially. Ultimately, very commonly, both legs are involved, although often asymmetrically. Although involvement may be as minimal as hyperactive reflexes or an extensor plantar response (Babinski sign), frequently severe spastic paraparesis develops. This is accompanied by abnormally brisk deep tendon reflexes, often to the point of clonus, especially at the ankles. Pathological spread of reflexes may be seen, often including tibioadductor and puboadductor reflexes.

Spasticity is very frequently present, more commonly in the legs than in the arms. Patients may indicate its existence with their complaints of stiffness, cramps, spasm, or pain. At times, the existence of spasticity may actually help an individual walk by providing increased stability to a patient whose legs are otherwise quite weak. In fact, it is not uncommon to encounter someone whose iliopsoas and hamstring muscles are very weak, perhaps 3/5 on the Medical Research Council grading system, but whose quadriceps remain with normal strength. The clinician must be wary of treating such patients too aggressively for spasticity, as this may actually diminish the patient's ability to walk. Conversely, when severe, spasticity may cause discomfort and pain, particularly in association with the production of flexor or extensor spasms, and may, additionally, lead to difficulties in personal hygiene (particularly because of adductor spasticity).

In the arms, corticospinal tract signs are again the most typical motor feature. However, it is rather common to see weakness predominate distally. In some instances, lower motor signs, with significant atrophy, are evident. These may be marked in the hand, with severe loss of function. This picture, which probably results from demyelination involving root fibers within or just as they exit the spinal cord, is sometimes referred to as a "trineural hand," as the clinical picture mimics one in which the radial, median, and ulnar nerves are all significantly affected.

Most of the clinical manifestations of corticospinal tract involvement result from lesions within the lateral columns of the spinal cord. However, the pyramidal tracts may be involved anywhere in their pathways, so that signs may result from lesions in the medullary pyramids, basis pontis, cerebral peduncles, internal capsules, or deep hemispheric white matter.

Hemiparetic patterns may appear, although much less commonly than those suggesting myelopathy. Occasionally, this appearance may be sudden in onset, implying a cerebrovascular etiology. In such cases, MRI typically provides evidence leading to the diagnosis of MS, with the clinically responsible lesion usually evident in the posterior limb of the internal capsule.

Somatosensory symptoms (Table 5.5)

As discussed above, sensory symptoms are the most common initial feature of MS and ultimately occur in 52–70% of patients. These variably described complaints most likely result from lesions in the myelinated posterior columns (fasciculi gracilis and cuneatus), rather than the spinothalamic tracts. In fact, when clinical signs, in addition to symptoms, are present these do tend to implicate the former long ascending tracts. These fibers mediate joint position and vibratory sensation. Impairment of the ability to perceive the vibration of a 128 Hz tuning fork, especially in the distal limbs (e.g. when the fork is applied to the big toe) is exceedingly common in established cases of MS and subtle reduction of this sensation may be one of the only detectable signs in patients with early disease.

Although less often encountered, diminished pain and temperature sensation or reduced sensitivity to light touch, reflecting involvement of the lateral and anterior spinothalamic tracts, respectively, are not uncommon. The patterns of altered sensitivity may again be extremely variable, but do at times indicate a spinal cord level. Sometimes the clinical picture mimics the Brown–Sequard syndrome of hemicord transection, demonstrating ipsilateral impairment of joint position and vibratory sense along with corticospinal tract weakness and contralateral impairment of pain and temperature sensation.

Table 5.5 Somatosensory symptoms

- Numbness
- Tingling
- Decreased feeling
- "Falling asleep"
- Tightness
- "Novocaine® wearing off"
- Like wearing a garment
- Like "walking on sand"
- Itching
- Burning
- Electricity
- Pain

Almost, but not quite, pathognomonic of MS is Lhermitte's sign (mis-termed as it is usually a symptom), in which the patient develops sudden sensations radiating down the spine or extremities, usually after flexing the neck.[25] The feelings are described most often as "like electricity," but other terms such as "vibration" or "buzzing" may be applied. The pattern of distribution of the sensation, as well as the maneuver that precipitates it, also vary. The phenomenon typically results from disease involving the posterior columns of the cervical spinal cord. While it may occur in other conditions affecting this structure, its occurrence is by far most common in MS.

MS is frequently, but mistakenly, considered to be a painless disorder. Regular encounters with patients in a clinical setting, as well as several systematic surveys, readily refute this notion.[26,27] The pain of MS may be a primary manifestation of the disease, or alternatively, may result from secondary consequences of the condition (Table 5.6).

Primary pain syndromes in MS include lancinating neuralgic complaints in a variety of sites. Best recognized is trigeminal neuralgia (discussed below), but similar sensations may occur elsewhere, including the extrem-ities. Another common type of pain is more chronic and persistent with a dysesthetic quality, often described as burning. The severity of these pains, which tend most often to occur in the distal lower extremities, can vary from mild annoyance to almost intolerable severity.

Spasticity is another source of pain. This sometimes produces abrupt paroxysmal pain, usually in association with occurrence of a sudden spasm (usually flexor, but sometimes extensor). However, more chronic aching limbs may also result.

Table 5.6 Pain syndromes

- Primary pain
  - Neuralgic pain
    - Trigeminal neuralgia
    - Other neuralgias
  - Dysesthetic pain
    - Most often burning (especially in legs)
    - Other dysesthesias
  - Radicular pain
  - Tonic seizures
  - Spasticity
    - Flexor spasms
    - Extensor spasms
  - Optic neuritis

- Secondary pain
  - Low back pain
  - Osteoporosis with fractures

Headache is a universal ailment that is most probably not overrepresented in the MS population. Occasionally, however, unusual headaches have occurred which appear to be a direct consequence of MS lesions. In one case, severe acute headache was associated with the development of a solitary new lesion in the periaqueductal gray area of the brainstem, a site from which stimulation with implanted electrodes has been shown to produce headache.[28] In another case, sudden severe headache accompanied by third nerve palsy suggested subarachnoid hemorrhage from a ruptured aneurysm.[29] Investigations revealed no evidence of bleeding or aneurysm, but cranial MRI showed more than 30 white matter lesions and cerebrospinal fluid contained oligoclonal bands resulting in the diagnosis of MS.

Pain can also result as a secondary consequence of MS lesions. For example, the weakness and abnormal gait commonly occurring in MS may lead to postural changes which predispose to low back pain, sometimes associated with radicular symptoms.

Even tertiary pain syndromes may occur in MS. Falls are a common consequence of the neurological deficits in MS and these are often associated with fractures. Furthermore, because of patients' diminished mobility, perhaps aggravated by recurrent steroid use, osteoporosis is a serious concern and another source of pain. Cosman et al noted a history of fractures in the absence of major trauma in 22% of MS patients, compared to only 2% of controls ($P < 0.002$).[30] Using dual X-ray absortiometry, these authors found that both women and men with MS experienced substantially more bone loss than controls during prospective follow-up of more than 2 years. Evidence is conflicting about the role of steroids, but low vitamin D intake and diminished exposure to sunlight appear to influence the development of osteoporosis in MS patients, already overrepresented by white women, the group generally at greatest risk for this bone disorder.

Visual pathway

As discussed above, optic neuritis is among the most frequent initial presentations of MS, occurring in 14–23% of case. However, even in the absence of frank acute optic neuritis, many patients will eventually demonstrate evidence of optic nerve involvement (Figure 5.5). Often visual acuity is measurably impaired, but sometimes only color vision is abnormal, detectable with Ishihara plates. Abnormal visual fields are frequently detectable by formal testing, though much less often evident at the bedside. The "swinging flashlight test" (Figure 5.6) often provides evidence of subtle optic nerve pathology by demonstrating an afferent pupillary defect (Marcus Gunn pupil).[31] Subclinical optic neuropathy may also be demonstrated electrophysiologically through visual evoked response testing (Figure 5.7).[32] Although optic nerve involvement, often

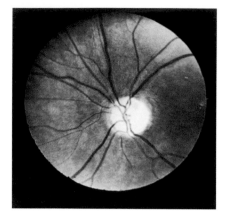

Figure 5.5
Pallor of the optic nerve head (optic atrophy) is a sequela of optic neuritis
(courtesy of Dr. Arthur Wolintz).

bilateral, is extremely common in MS, fortunately blindness is relatively infrequent.

Almost any imaginable visual field defect may be encountered in MS, though central or paracentral scotomata are most characteristic (Figure 5.1). Bilateral homonymous visual field defects, as well as quadrantanopsias, occur, sometimes associated with anatomically appropriate lesions demonstrable on MRI.

Olfaction and gustation

MS patients rarely offer spontaneous complaints of disturbances of smell or taste or even acknowledge the symptom on direct inquiry. However, recent studies using forced choice testing (University of Pennsylvania Smell Identification Test) demonstrated abnormalities in as many as 38.5% of patients.[33] High scores on the test (normal olfaction) have been negatively correlated with the number of lesions detected on MRI in the inferior frontal and temporal lobes, areas associated with the sense of smell.

Very rare case reports have documented presentation of MS with disturbances of the sense of taste. Hemiageusia has been reported, antedating the occurrence of other brainstem manifestations, and associated with MR demonstration of medullary abnormality.[34]

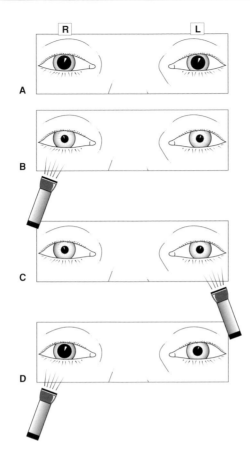

Figure 5.6
Swinging flashlight test demonstrating afferent pupillary defect in right eye.
(A) Pupils at medium size in ambient light (test is best performed in a darkened
room). (B) Flashlight beamed at right eye results in both direct and consensual
pupillary constriction. (C) Flashlight beamed at unaffected left eye again elicits
direct and consensual pupillary constriction. (D) Flashlight swung back to side of
afferent pupillary defect now elicits pupillary dilatation because light stimulus is
perceived as less intense than when beam was aimed at normal left eye.

Cerebellar manifestations

Although less common than other symptoms in the initial presentation
of MS, evidence of cerebellar dysfunction is ultimately quite frequent,
occurring in as many as 50% of patients. This may be manifest as gait
ataxia, suggesting involvement of the midline vermis. Alternatively,
cerebellar hemispheric pathology may produce symptoms in the ipsi-

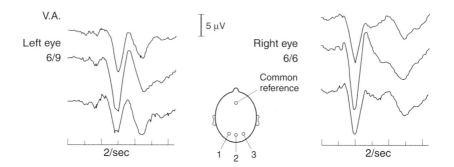

Figure 5.7
Visual evoked response testing demonstrates the characteristic delayed latency of the p100 peak in the left eye.

lateral extremities. Typical cerebellar signs, including intention tremor, dysmetria (seen on finger-to-nose testing in the arms and heel-knee-shin testing in the legs), dysdiadochokinesia (clumsy rapid alternating movements), and, less commonly, hypotonia, may all be found. Sometimes violent tremors on attempted movement, so-called rubral tremors, are encountered and may be extremely disabling. Cerebellar involvement also produces dysarthria. The classic speech disturbance, referred to as scanning speech, is characterized by a particular rhythm and cadence in which each word or syllable is given nearly equal emphasis; it is actually much less common than impaired articulatory agility.[35] The latter type of dysarthria can be readily demonstrated by asking the patient to repeat the sequence pah-tah-kah in rapid succession.

Brainstem disturbances

A wide variety of abnormalities of brainstem function occur, but disturbances of extraocular motility are most regularly encountered. Nystagmus is extremely common, most often of the gaze evoked horizontal type.[2,3] Similarly, vertical – usually upbeat – nystagmus may be seen. Other types of nystagmus, including rotatory, downbeat, and mixed forms, occur, as well as wilder ocular gyrations at times. Although the nystagmus is frequently asymptomatic, patients may complain of jumping vision (oscillopsia), simply blurred vision, or double vision.

Internuclear ophthalmoplegia (INO) is among the most characteristic abnormalities in MS (Figure 5.8). A result of a lesion in the medial longitudinal fasciculus (MLF), it may occur either unilaterally or bilaterally.[36,37] In classic form, on lateral gaze the eye fails to adduct on the side of the MLF lesion, while the contralateral abducting eye develops horizontal nystagmus. The eyes are not displaced at rest and frequently the patient has no visual symptoms, although double vision may be reported. Incomplete forms, sometimes simply with dissociated nystagmus, are common.[38,39] In a young person, INO, especially when bilateral, is virtually pathognomonic of MS.

Because lesions can occur anywhere along the pathways for extraocular movements, a variety of other abnormalities may result. These include horizontal (sometimes bilateral) and vertical gaze paresis, the one-and-a-half syndrome (in which a horizontal gaze paresis to one side is combined with an adduction failure to the other side),[40,41] dysfunction of individual muscles, and skew deviation. These signs may or may not be accompanied by visual symptoms, although individual muscle paresis typically causes diplopia.

In addition to the dysarthria decribed above as a consequence of cerebellar disease, other speech disturbances may result from brainstem lesions. Explosive, poorly modulated speech is characteristic of pseudo-

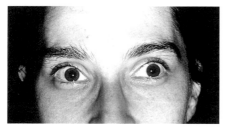

(A)

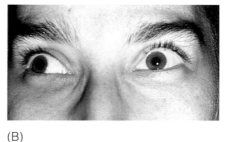

(B)

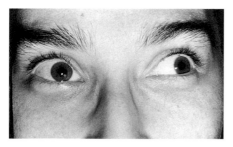

(C)

Figure 5.8
Patient with bilateral internuclear ophthalmoplegia. (A) At straightahead gaze, eyes are essentially midline. (B) On right lateral gaze, the right eye fully abducts, but the left eye does not adduct, indicating a lesion of the left median longitudinal fasciculus (MLF). (C) On left lateral gaze, the left eye fully abducts, but the right eye fails to adduct, indicating a lesion of the right MLF (courtesy of Dr. Arthur Wolintz).

bulbar palsy, a syndrome resulting from bilateral corticobulbar tract lesions.[35] Other features of the syndrome include facial biparesis, hyperactive gag reflexes, poor palatal movement, dysphagia, and slow tongue movements. Sometimes nasal speech results from involvement of cranial nerves IX and X.

Facial paresis as a result of involvement of corticobulbar tract is common, but sometimes peripheral palsy, exactly resembling Bell's palsy, occurs.[42] Presumably this results from demyelination of the facial nerve within the brainstem.

Other facial movement abnormalities also occur. Facial myokymia, or undulating, wave-like fascicular twitching, is characteristic of MS.[43] This usually begins or is limited to the orbicularis oculi muscles and may persist for days. Blepharospasm has been described,[44] usually in association with other brainstem signs, and hemifacial spasm also occurs.

Disturbances of the auditory system, while relatively uncommon in MS, are not rare.[45] Unilateral or bilateral hearing loss may occur. In fact, when patients present with isolated hearing loss, cranial MRI not infrequently reveals unexpected evidence of MS. Tinnitus is an occasional complaint of MS patients.

Symptoms of vestibular system involvement, by contrast, are quite frequent in MS. Vertigo usually occurs as part of an acute exacerbation, often associated with other signs of brainstem dysfunction, especially eye movement abnormalities. However, vague complaints of dizziness seem to be present in many chronically affected patients. Intractable hiccups have also been rarely reported.[46,47]

Gait disturbances

Eventually gait abnormalities become one of the most disabling aspects of MS for many patients. The problem stems most often from spastic paraparesis. If the weakness predominates on one side, the gait may be characterized by circumduction of one leg. When bilateral weakness involves proximal muscles, the gait may have a waddling quality. Often, in the face of significant loss of strength in the large leg muscles, gait is preserved because of the existence of spasticity. This tends to be prominent in the leg extensors, whose strength is often well preserved in the typical corticospinal pattern of weakness. Antispasticity medication must be administered cautiously because too much reduction in tone will result in further deterioration of gait. Another manifestation of pyramidal tract weakness common in MS is foot drop, which may be helped by the use of an ankle–foot orthosis.

Ataxia, although less common than spastic paresis, is another frequent cause of abnormal gait. This is usually a result of cerebellar disease, but may, on occasion, occur with severe proprioceptive disturbance resulting from lesions of the posterior columns of the spinal cord. Vestibular dysfunction and abnormalities of vision may also contribute to difficulty walking.

Cognitive and psychiatric disturbances

Patients spontaneously voice complaints about difficulties with memory and concentration with very high frequency. Indeed, formal neuropsychological testing confirms the existence of cognitive problems in a great many patients and far more often than bedside clinical examination reveals.[48] Fortunately, the abnormalities are usually not severe and are most notable in attention and concentration, memory, and conceptual reasoning-problem solving. This is a pattern most typically associated with subcortical lesions. Frank dementia does occur at times. The presence and severity of cognitive impairment do not correlate well with either duration or severity of illness, but recent studies have shown a relationship to the extent and distribution of MRI lesions.[49] Aphasia and neglect have been reported very rarely.[50,51]

Euphoria was widely described as a feature of MS in earlier literature. In fact, depression is far more common, affecting as many as 75% of patients during the course of the illness. This is usually mild and readily amenable to treatment, but major depression may also occur.[52-54] What has often been mistaken for euphoria (an actual aberration of mood) is the inability to inhibit emotional expression, usually resulting from subcortical forebrain lesions. This condition results in both "inappropriate" laughing and crying.[55] Sometimes apparent euphoria seems to occur in patients with prominent cognitive decline.

Rarely other psychotic conditions, resembling schizophrenia or other delusional syndromes, occur. This may reflect more disease in the temporal lobe periventricular areas.[56,57]

Fatigue and sleep

Among the most regularly encountered (up to 90% of patients), and at times perplexing, symptoms in MS is fatigue.[58,59] While this is often increased at the time of an acute exacerbation, fatigue is often persistently present. The complaint of fatigue should prompt further exploration by the clinician, for many different circumstances may lead to the symptom (Table 5.7).

Of course, MS patients are certainly no more resistant than unaffected individuals to the normal causes of fatigue such as overwork and inadequate sleep. Because MS patients often have muscle weakness and gait abnormalities, they may become more readily exhausted by exercise or walking which exceeds their limits. As indicated above, depression commonly afflicts people with MS and fatigue, as well as sleep disturbance –

Table 5.7 Fatigue

"Ordinary"
 • Overwork
 • Inadequate sleep

Pathological
 • Secondary to muscle weakness
 • Secondary to conduction failure
 • Secondary to depression
 • Unique MS fatigue (overwhelming sense of enervation)

Secondary to medications

most typically early morning awakening – may be a symptom of this psychiatric syndrome.

However, a unique form of fatigue also appears to occur commonly in MS patients. This is a severe feeling of enervation, often preventing a patient from carrying out ordinary work, family, or social obligations.[60] Medication may help this particular type of fatigue, but first it is necessary that other lifestyle modifications be explored.

Recently, disturbances of sleep have also been noted to be much more common in MS patients than in the general population.[61] This may be associated with depression or may result from excessive awakenings, perhaps due to nocturia. Restless legs or periodic limb movements of sleep have been reported to occur with increased frequency in MS patients.

Bladder, bowel, and sexual disturbances

Another cause of disabling symptoms in MS is urinary bladder dysfunction, with disturbances of micturition or defecation ultimately affecting as many as 80% of patients (Table 5.8). Urinary frequency and urgency are the most frequent complaints, the latter sometimes accompanied by incontinence. Conversely, hesitancy may occur and, on occasion, frank urinary retention. History alone does not reliably provide an accurate

Table 5.8 Bladder dysfunction

 • Failure to store
 • Failure to empty
 • Combination of failure to store and failure to empty

guide to the nature of the physiological abnormality.[62,63] However, often the only investigation necessary before initiation of treatment is a measure of the residual urine volume after the well hydrated patient voids. Disturbances of micturition may be characterized as failure to store, failure to empty, or a combination of both.[62,63] Frequently in MS contraction of the urinary bladder is accompanied by contraction of the external urethral sphincter, rather than the appropriate relaxation (Figure 5.9). This condition, known as detrusor-external sphincter dyssynergia, may then lead to urinary retention and a predisposition to infection. Particularly in males, vesicoureteral reflux may develop with the threat of hydronephrosis and potential renal failure.

Bowel dysfunction, though less socially disabling than urinary symptoms, is also very frequent.[64,65] Constipation has a prevalence rate of 39–53% and may result from autonomic dysfunction, abnormal rectal function, or even intussuception.[64,66,67] Patients with urinary frequency and urgency often decrease their fluid intake in a misguided attempt to relieve these symptoms, with the resultant consequence of aggravated constipation. Fecal incontinence is also surprisingly common in MS, with 51% of patients in one series experiencing incontinence at least once in the preceding 3 months and 25% at least weekly.[65]

Impaired sexual function is often present, particularly in patients with urinary symptoms. Men commonly experience erectile dysfunction, but may at times have disturbances of ejaculation.[68] By contrast, women most often complain of difficulty achieving orgasm, sometimes related to diminished genital sensitivity.[69] Inadequate lubrication may also occur. Both men and women may also complain of diminished libido, which may be a direct or indirect consequence of the disease.

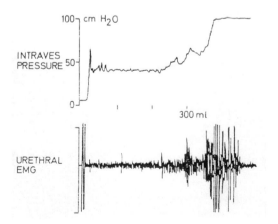

Figure 5.9

Detrusor sphincter dyssynergia. Instead of relaxing when the bladder contracts, the urethral sphincter also contracts, interfering with the expulsion of urine.

Table 5.9 Paroxysmal symptoms

- Trigeminal neuralgia (and other neuralgias)
- Tonic "seizures"
- Paroxysmal dysarthria
- Paroxysmal itching
- Hemifacial spasm
- Sudden loss of muscle tone
- Paroxysmal aphasia
- Paroxysmal kinesogenic choreoathetosis
- Lhermitte's sign

Paroxysmal symptoms

Sudden, brief stereotyped symptoms and signs are a well recognized phenomenon in MS (Table 5.9).[70,71] Most widely described have been tonic "seizures".[72–75] These are not seizures in the epileptic sense, but rather sudden dystonic posturing of part of the body, usually the hand or arm. These attacks typically last between 30 seconds and 2 minutes and may be painful. The events may occur infrequently or many times a day, but tend to cluster over weeks to months. Lesions in a variety of sites, including the basal ganglia, internal capsule, thalamus, cerebral peduncle, and cervical spinal cord, have been associated with tonic seizures.

Probably the most common paroxysmal symptom is trigeminal neuralgia.[76,77] This clinical syndrome of lancinating pain, most often in the second division of the nerve, is generally indistinguishable from that occurring in individuals without MS. The symptom does tend to occur at a younger age and is more commonly bilateral in those with the demyelinating disease.[77] Similar neuralgic pains may occur in other parts of the body.

Other symptoms of this nature include paroxysmal dysarthria (with or without accompanying brainstem signs), paroxysmal itching, and hemifacial spasm. Patients may also report sudden loss of muscle tone in the lower extremities

Movement disorders

Although decidedly uncommon, examples of unusual movement disorder have occurred in MS. Hemiballismus was described in a rare case of infantile MS. Kinesigenic dystonia and paroxysmal kinesigenic choreoathetosis have each been reported as the initial presentation of MS.[78] Segmental myoclonus resulting from spinal cord lesions may occur[79] and trismus has been described.

Autonomic disturbances

Autonomic disturbances, other than the frequent bladder and bowel dysfunction, probably occur much more often than recognized. Particularly common are coldness or discoloration of the legs or feet, but abnormal sweating has also been described.[80] Recently, several patients have been reported with significant hypothermia occurring during acute relapses.[81] Most of these patients were severely disabled and had other evidence of brainstem lesions during the exacerbations. Rarely disturbed respiratory patterns occur and respiratory failure may result from bilateral diaphragmatic paralysis.

Summary

Multiple sclerosis is a disease affecting people, women much more often than men, in the prime of their lives. It is progressive in the vast majority of patients, with gait impairment, urinary incontinence, and severe fatigue the most frequently disabling symptoms. The clinical manifestations are protean and attacks develop unpredictably. The apparent capriciousness of disease exacerbation, coupled with the often rapid appearance of disabling neurological symptoms, greatly taxes the coping skills of patients even in the early stages of the illness. Hopefully the availability of new immunomodulatory treatments, increasingly administered early in the course of the illness, will ultimately result in a much more benign course for many patients.

References

1. Kurtzke JF. Clinical manifestations of multiple sclerosis. In: Vinken PJ, Bruyn GW, eds. Multiple sclerosis and other demyelinating diseases. Amsterdam: North Holland; 1970: 161–216.

2. McAlpine D. Symptoms and signs. In: McAlpine D, Lumsden CE, Acheson ED, eds. Multiple sclerosis: a reappraisal. Baltimore: Williams and Wilkins; 1972: 132–196.

3. Muller R. Studies on disseminated sclerosis with special reference to symptomatology, course and prognosis. Acta Med Scand Suppl 1949; 222:1–214.

4. Lublin FD, Reingold SC. Defining the clinical course of multiple sclerosis: results of an international survey. Neurology 1996; 46:907–911.

5. Interferon beta-1b multiple sclerosis study group. Interferon beta-1b is effective in relapsing-remitting multiple sclerosis: I. Clinical results of a multicenter, randomized, double-blind, placebo-controlled trial. Neurology 1993; 43:655–661.

6. Jacobs LD, Cookfair DL, Rudick RA, et al. Intramuscular interferon beta-1a for disease progression in relapsing multiple sclerosis. Ann Neurol 1996; 39:285–294.

7. Johnson KP, Brooks BR, Cohen JA, et al. Copolymer 1 reduces the relapse rate and improves disability in relapsing-remitting multiple sclerosis: results of phase III multicenter, double-blind, placebo-controlled trial. Neurology 1995; 45:1268–1276.

8. Weinshenker BG, Bass B, Rice GPB, et al. The natural history of multiple sclerosis: a geographically-based study. I. Clinical course and disability. Brain 1989; 112:133–146.

9. Confavreux C, Hutchinson M, Hours MM, Cortinovis-Tourniaire P,

Moreau T. Rate of pregnancy-related relapse in multiple sclerosis. Pregnancy in Multiple Sclerosis Group. N Engl J Med 1998; 339:285–291.

10. Kurtzke JF. Rating neurologic impairment in multiple sclerosis: an expanded disability status scale (EDSS). Neurology 1983; 33:1444–1452.

11. Miller A, Drexler E, Keilson M, et al. Spontaneous stabilization in patients with chronic progressive MS. Neurology 1988; 38(suppl 1):194.

12. Wynn DR, Rodriguez M, O'Fallon WM, et al. A reappraisal of the epidemiology of multiple sclerosis in Olmsted County, Minnesota. Neurology 1990; 40:780–786.

13. Kurtzke JF, Beebe GW, Nagler B, et al. Studies on the natural history of multiple sclerosis. 5. Long-term survival in young men. Arch Neurol 1970; 22:215–225.

14. Panitch HS, Hirsch RL, Schindler J, Johnson KP. Treatment of multiple sclerosis with gamma interferon: exacerbations associated with activation of the immune system. Neurology 1987; 37:1097–1102.

15. Banford CR, Sibley WA, Thies C, et al. Trauma as an etiologic and aggravating factor in multiple sclerosis. Neurology 1981; 31:1229–1234.

16. Goodin DS, Ebers GC, Johnson KP, et al. The relationship of MS to physical trauma and psychological stress. Report of the Therapeutics and Technology Assessment Subcommittee of the American Academy of Neurology. Neurology 1999; 52:1737–1745.

17. Nispeanu P, Korczyn A. A psychological stress as risk factor for exacerbations in multiple sclerosis. Neurology 1993; 43:1311–1312.

18. Birk K, Smeltzer SKFC, et al. The effect of pregnancy in multiple sclerois. Neurology 1988; 38(suppl 1):237.

19. Frith JA, McLeod JG. Pregnancy and multiple sclerosis. J Neurol Neurosurg Psychiatry 1988; 51:495–498.

20. Korn-Lubetzki I, Kahana E, Cooper G, et al. Activity of multiple sclerosis during pregnancy and puerperium. Ann Neurol 1984; 15:229–231.

21. Thomason DS, Nelson LM, Burns A. The effects of pregnancy in multiple sclerosis: a retrospective study. Neurology 1986; 36:1097–1099.

22. Confavreux C, Hutchinson M, Hours MM, et al. Rate of pregnancy-related relapse in multiple sclerosis. N Engl J Med 1998; 339:285–291.

23. Berdru P, Theys P, D'Hooghe MB, et al. Pregnancy in multiple sclerosis: the influence on long-term disability. Clin Neurol Neurosurg 1994; 96:38–41.

24. Runmarker B, Anderson O. Pregnancy is associated with a lower risk of onset and a better prognosis in multiple sclerosis. Brain 1995; 118:253–261.

25. Lhermitte J, Bollak P, Nichas M. Les douleurs a type de decharge electrique consecutives a la flexion cephalique dans la sclerose en plaques. Rev Neurol 1924; 42:56–62.

26. Clifford DB, Trotter JL. Pain in multiple sclerosis. Arch Neurol 1984; 41:1270–1272.

27. Moulin DE, Foley KM, Ebers GC. Pain syndromes in multiple sclerosis. Neurology 1988; 38:1830–1834.

28. Haas DC, Kent PF, Friedman DL. Headache caused by a single lesion of multiple sclerosis in the periaqueductal gray area. Headache 1993; 33:452–455.

29. Galer BS, Lipton RB, Weinstein S, et al. Apoplectic headache and

oculomotor palsy: an unusual presentation of multiple sclerosis. Neurology 1990; 40:1465–1466.

30. Cosman F, Nieves J, Komar L, et al. Fracture history and bone loss in patients with multiple sclerosis. Neurology 1998; 51:1161–1165.

31. Stanley JA, Baise G. The swinging flashlight test to detect minimal optic neuropathy. Arch Ophthalmol 1968; 80:769–771.

32. Halliday AM, McDonald WI, Mushin J. Delayed visual evoked response in optic neuritis. Lancet 1972; i:982–985.

33. Doty RL, Li C, Mannon LJ, et al. Olfactory dysfunction in multiple sclerosis. N Engl J Med 1997; 336:1918–1919.

34. Pascual-Leone A, Altafullah I, Dhura A. Hemiageusia: an unusual presentation of multiple sclerosis. J Neurol Neurosurg Psychiatry 1991; 54:657.

35. Dailey FL, Brown JR, Goldstein FJ. Dysarthria in multiple sclerosis. Speech Hear Res 1972; 15:229–245.

36. Bender MB, Weinstein EA. Dissociated monocular nystagmus with paresis of horizontal ocular movements. Arch Ophthalmol 1939; 21:266–272.

37. Wilson SAK. Case of disseminated sclerosis with weakness of each internal rectus and nystagmus on lateral deviation limited to the outer eye. Brain 1906; 29:298.

38. Cogan DG. Internuclear ophthalmoplegia, typical and atypical. Arch Ophthalmol 1970; 1970:583–589.

39. Muri R, Meienberg O. The clinical spectrum of internuclear ophthalmoplegia in multiple sclerosis. Arch Neurol 1985; 42:851–855.

40. Fisher CM. Some neuro-ophthalmological observations. J Neurol Neurosurg Psychiatry 1967; 30:383–392.

41. Wall M, Wray SH. The one-and-a-half syndrome – a unilateral disorder of the pontine tegmentum: a study of 20 cases and review of the literature. Neurology 1983; 33:971–980.

42. Ivers RR, Goldstein NP. Multiple sclerosis: a current appraisal of symptoms and signs. Mayo Clin Proc 1963; 338:457–466.

43. Andermann F, Cosgrove JBR, Lloyd-Smith DL, et al. Facial myokymia in multiple sclerosis. Brain 1961; 84:31–44.

44. Jankovic J, Patel SC. Blepharospasm associated with brainstem lesions. Neurology 1983; 33:1237–1240.

45. Daugherty WT, Lederman RJ, Nodar RH, et al. Hearing loss in multiple sclerosis. Arch Neurol 1983; 40:33–35.

46. Birkhead R, Friedman HJ. Hiccups and vomiting as initial manifestations of multiple sclerosis. J Neurol Neurosurg Psychiatry 1987; 50:232–233.

47. McFarlin DA, Susac JO. Hoquet diabolique: intractable hiccups as a manifestation of multiple sclerosis. Neurology 1979; 29:797–801.

48. Rao SM, Hammeke TA, McQuillen MP, et al. Memory disturbance in chronic progressive multiple sclerosis. Arch Neurol 1984; 41:625–631.

49. Franklin GM, Heaton RK, Nelson LM, et al. Correlation of neuropsychological and MRI findings in chronic progressive multiple sclerosis. Neurology 1988; 38:1826–18.

50. Achiron A, Ziv I, Djaldetti R, et al. Aphasia in multiple sclerosis: clinical and radiologic correlations. Neurology 1992; 42:2195–2197.

51. Graff-Radford NR, Rizzo M. Neglect in a patient with multiple sclerosis. Eur Neurol 1987; 26:100–103.

52. Cottrell SS, Wilson SAK. The affec-

tive symptomatology of dissemi-nated sclerosis. J Neurol Psychopathol 1926; 7:1–30.

53. Schiffer RB. The spectrum of depression in multiple sclerosis: an approach for clinical manage-ment. Arch Neurol 1987; 44:596–599.

54. Whitlock FA, Siskind MM. Depression as a major symptom of multiple sclerosis. J Neurol Neurosurg Psychiatry 1980; 43:861–865.

55. Schiffer RB, Herndon RM, Rudick RA. Treatment of pathologic laugh-ing and weeping with amitriptyline. N Engl J Med 1985; 312: 1480–1482.

56. Feinstein A, duBoulay G, Ron MA. Psychotic illness in multiple sclero-sis. A clinical and magnetic reso-nance imaging study. Br J Psychiatry 1992; 161:680–685.

57. Honer WG, Hurwitz, Li DKB. Temporal lobe involvement in mul-tiple sclerosis patients with psychi-atric disorders. Arch Neurol 1987; 44:187–190.

58. Freal JE, Kraft GH, Coryell SK. Symptomatic fatigue in multiple sclerosis. Arch Phys Med Rehabil 1984; 65:135–138.

59. Murray TJ. Amantadine therapy for fatigue in multiple sclerosis. Can J Neurol Sci 1985; 12:251–254.

60. Krupp L, La Rocca NG, Muir-Nash J, et al. Fatigue severity scale. Neurology 1988; 38:99–100.

61. Clark CM, Fleming JA, Li D, et al. Sleep disturbances, depression, and lesion site in patients with mul-tiple sclerosis. Arch Neurol 1992; 49:641–643.

62. Blaivas JG, Acheson ED. Management of bladder dys-function in multiple sclerosis. Neurology 1980; 30:12–18.

63. Blaivas JG, Barbalias GA. Detrusor-external sphincter dyssynergia in men with multiple

sclerosis: an ominous urologic condition. J Urol 1984; 131:91–94.

64. Fowler CJ, Henry MM. Gastro-intestinal dysfunction in multiple sclerosis. Int Mult Scler J 1999; 6:59–61.

65. Hinds JP, Eidelman BH, Wald A. Prevalence of bowel dysfunction in multiple sclerosis: a population survey. Gastroenterology 1990; 98:1538–1542.

66. Chia YW, Fowler C, Kamm M, et al. Prevalence of bowel dysfunction in patients with multiple sclerosis and bladder dysfunction. J Neurol 1995; 242:105–108.

67. Nordenbo A, Andersen J, Andersen J. Disturbances of ano-rectal function in multiple sclero-sis. J Neurol 1996; 243:445–451.

68. Vas CJ. Sexual impotence and some autonomic disturbances in men with multiple sclerosis. Acta Neurol Scand 1969; 45:166–183.

69. Lundberg PO. Sexual dysfunction in female patients with multiple sclerosis. Int Rehabil Med 1981; 3:32–34.

70. Miller A. In: Burks JS, Johnson KP, eds. Multiple sclerosis, diagnosis, medical management, and reha-bilitation. New York: Demos; 2000: 377–384.

71. Twomey JA, Espir MLE. Paroxysmal symptoms as the first manifestations of multiple sclero-sis. J Neurol Neurosurg Psychiatry 1980; 43:296–304.

72. Berger JR, Sheremata WA, Melamed E. Paroxysmal dystonia as the initial manifestation of multi-ple sclerosis. Arch Neurol 1984; 41:747–750.

73. Heath PD, Nightingale S. Clusters of tonic spasms as an initial mani-festation of multiple sclerosis. Ann Neurol 1982; 12:494–495.

74. Joynt RJ, Green D. Tonic seizures as a manifestation of multiple scle-

rosis. Arch Neurol 1962; 6:293–299.

75. Matthews WB. Tonic seizures in disseminated sclerosis. Brain 1958; 81:193–206.

76. Brisman R. Trigeminal neuralgia in multiple sclerosis. Arch Neurol 1987; 44:379–381.

77. Hooge JP, Redekop WK. Trigeminal neuralgia in multiple sclerosis. Neurology 1995; 45:1294–1296.

78. Roos RA, Wintzen AR, Vielvoye G, et al. Paroxysmal kinesigenic choreoathetosis as presenting symptom of multiple sclerosis. J Neurol Neurosurg Psychiatry 1991; 54:657–658.

79. Kapoor R, Brown P, Thompson PD, et al. Propriospinal myoclonus in multiple sclerosis. J Neurol Neurosurg Psychiatry 1992; 55:1086–1088.

80. Cartlidge NEF. Autonomic function in multiple sclerosis. Brain 1972; 95:661–664.

81. White KD, Scoones DJ, Newman PK. Hypothermia in multiple sclerosis. J Neurol Neurosurg Psychiatry 1996; 61:369–375.

6
MRI in MS

Overview

Magnetic resonance imaging (MRI) is a relatively modern technique, with the first human study conducted in 1977. MRI has become the major paraclinical test for MS. Most importantly, it provides information on multiple disease dimensions (Table 6.1).[1] MRI offers a number of advantages over alternative neuroimaging techniques such as plain X-ray, computerized tomography, radionuclide scanning, positron emission tomography, or single photon emission computed tomography (Table 6.2). It is safe, and can be repeated multiple times. In relapsing and secondary progressive patients (85% of the MS population), serial brain MRI remains the best marker of disease activity.[2] Although MRI lesions are more sensitive than specific for MS, new techniques currently under evaluation are likely to improve on disease specificity.

Although both brain and spinal cord MRI are useful in MS, brain MRI is obtained much more often because it detects approximately ten times the number of lesions seen in spinal cord. MRI can visualize the central nerv-

Table 6.1 Role of MRI in MS.

- Diagnosis
- Natural history studies
- Disease pathogenesis studies
- Prognosis/correlation studies
- Clinical trials/outcome measures

Table 6.2 Advantages of MRI for neuroimaging.

- Noninvasive
- No radiation exposure
- No identified safety concerns from magnetic field exposure
- Can be repeated multiple times
- Can image in any plane without loss of resolution
- Very sensitive for lesion detection
- No problems with bony artifact
- Provides good detail of difficult areas, such as brainstem and spinal cord

ous system (CNS) in three basic orthogonal planes, axial (transverse), sagittal, and coronal, without moving the patient (Figure 6.1). It can also image in any oblique orientation.

MRI is carried out with or without contrast. At the current time there are three gadolinium chelates, all equally effective. Gadolinium-diethylenetri-amine pentaacetic acid (Gd-DPTA) is the standard intravenous contrast.

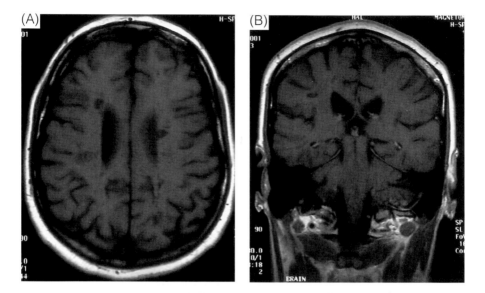

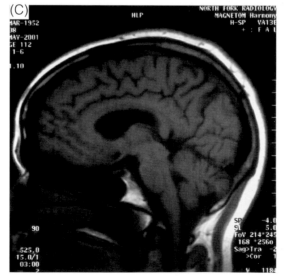

Figure 6.1
Examples of axial (A), coronal (B) and sagittal (C) MRI scans.

Contrast enhancing lesions identify areas where there is a major blood–brain barrier breakdown.

This chapter will first review basic MRI characteristics, then discuss currently available techniques, and finally consider the varied role of MRI in evaluating MS.

Background

MRI uses the principle of nuclear magnetic resonance – that certain mobile protons will line up in a magnetic field. Approximately 90% of the human body is water, and current MRI relies on abundant hydrogen protons. Protons will align either parallel or antiparallel to an applied magnetic field. The orientation of this lineup can be influenced by parameters such as temperature and field strength. As protons flip back to return to their initial alignment, they generate a signal which induces an electric current in a receiver coil. This ultimately creates the MRI image, based on data reconstructed according to the spatial distribution of the signal.

MRI requires a patient to be placed into a strong magnetic field and subjected to a radiofrequency pulse. Not everyone can tolerate this. Because of the magnetic field exposure, patients with metallic implants, devices, or foreign bodies (such as cardiac pacemaker, aneurysm clip, metallic rods/screws) cannot be scanned. MRI involves insertion into a rather noisy, dark, and enclosed machine. Very large individuals may not be able to fit into the machine, and claustrophobic individuals, pediatric patients, emotionally disturbed individuals, or those in extreme pain may need to be sedated. For some large or claustrophobic patients, open machines may be required. Open MRI is inferior to closed MRI for evaluating MS, but is preferable to no study.

Net magnetization refers to the sum of the contributions of all the magnetic moments of the protons.[3] Net magnetization has two major components: longitudinal (along the direction of the static magnetic field) and transverse (orthogonal to the magnetic field). As protons flip back to their original alignment, they provide two distinct relaxation components, T1 and T2 (Table 6.3). Both of these components give unique information about the protons within the tissue being studied. Differences in relaxation rates (T1/T2) are translated into a gray scale to produce optical contrasts. Image contrasts can be made T1 or T2 weighted (T1W or T2W).[4]

Basic MRI technical issues such as magnet strength, voxel size, and slice thickness all affect spatial resolution. Standard high field magnets are 1.5 tesla (T). Stronger (3 and 4 T) magnets are used in research studies to provide better resolution, and even higher fields are available at a few centers. Signal intensity increases with field strength. Voxel volume is manipulated by slice thickness and matrix dimensions; the smaller the volume, the more highly defined is the region of interest. Slice thickness is typically 3 mm, but can range up to 5 mm, or as low as 1 mm. Signal to noise ratio increases with voxel size, and decreases with thinner slices. Slices can be contiguous, or have a gap. Sensitivity for lesion detection increases with contiguous slices.

Table 6.3 Magnetization relaxation components.

- T1 time constant
  - Describes longitudinal relaxation
  - Time when 63% of original magnetization is reached
  - Spin–lattice relaxation
  - 300–2000 ms
- T2 time constant
  - Describes transverse component
  - Time when transverse magnetization decreases to 37% of original value
  - Spin–spin relaxation
  - 30–150 ms (T2 always ≤ T1)

Conventional techniques

MRI involves several standard pulse sequences (Table 6.4). Spin echo sequences use distinct repetition times (TR) and echo times (TE) to produce T2W, proton density (PD), or T1W images. TR is the time interval necessary for longitudinal magnetization to occur after a radiofrequency pulse perturbation. TE is the time from the original radiofrequency pulse to the

Table 6.4 Conventional MRI sequences/techniques.

- Spin echo sequences
  - T2 weighted (T2W) images
    - Long TE (> 60 ms)
    - Long TR (>2000 ms)
  - Proton density (PD) images
    - Short TE (< 30 ms)
    - Long TR (> 2000 ms)
  - T1 weighted (T1W) images
    - Short TE < 30 ms)
    - Short TR (< 800 ms)
    - Used for contrast studies

- Fast sequences
  - Fast spin echo
  - Turbogradient spin echo
  - Echoplanar imaging

- Inversion recovery sequences (heavily T1W)
  - Fluid attenuated inversion recovery (FLAIR)
  - Short tau inversion recovery (STIR)

TE, echo time; TR, repetition time.

peak of the re-emitted echo. Examples of different spin echo sequences are shown in Figure 6.2.

On T2 images CSF appears bright (hyperintense), while normal gray and white matter are dark. Virtually all pathological processes produce increased water content within cells and surrounding tissue, so that

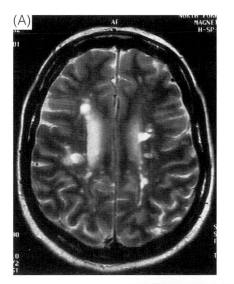
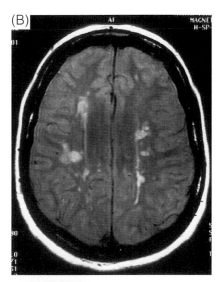
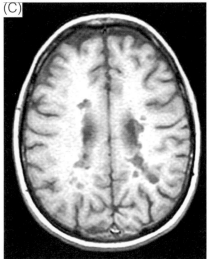

Figure 6.2
The T2 weighted image (A) and the proton density image (B) from the same patient show many lesions, predominantly in the periventricular areas, that appear as increased signal (white). The T1 weighted image (C) from another patient shows several lesions of decreased signal ("black holes").

abnormal tissue appears bright on T2 MRI. Although this sequence is quite sensitive to detect lesions, it is not very specific. Heterogeneous pathologies (edema, inflammation, demyelination, remyelination, gliosis, axon loss) produce identical appearing hyperintense signal. There are certain neuroanatomic areas where T2 MRI is relatively insensitive. Lesions adjacent to CSF are not imaged well, and lesions in the cortex, subcortex, and periventricular regions are underestimated. This can be solved by use of inversion recovery sequences (see below). T2 MRI is used to measure total lesion burden in the brain, also referred to as lesion load or burden of disease. T2 is also used to detect new or enlarging brain lesions. There is no method of dating T2 lesions, which can range from days to years in age. T2 brain lesions become more common over age 50 even in healthy controls, presumably due to microvascular changes. This is in striking contrast to spinal cord MRI, where intramedullary lesions do not occur with aging. In relapsing and early secondary progressive MS, most new T2 lesions reflect acute inflammatory events.

PD is another form of spin echo, usually considered along with T2. It involves a short T1. On PD CSF is dark, white matter is light, and gray matter is even lighter. MS lesions appear white, similar to T2 imaging.

T1 images use a short repetition time (TR 450–700 ms) and short echo time (TE 5–20 ms). CSF has very little signal and appears dark, while gray matter is intermediate, and white matter is light. Lesions which are hyperintense on T2 and PD MRI are either hypointense on T1 (so-called black holes), or are isointense and therefore invisible. A T1 black hole has a lower signal intensity than surrounding white matter (equal to or lower than gray matter). The degree of hypointensity will be influenced by MRI sequence selection, and whether the T1 gradient is mild or extreme. The pathological changes associated with T1 hypointense lesions involve axon loss and reduction in axon density, extracellular edema, and myelin disruption. In general, the more hypointense the lesion, the more destructive the tissue changes.[5] T1 hypointense lesions are common supratentorially, unusual in the posterior fossa, and not reported in the spinal cord. They are more common in primary and secondary progressive patients than in relapsing patients. A recent study found higher median T1 lesions in male vs. female primary progressive patients.[6]

MS T1 lesions vary. Early active lesions are iso or minimally hypointense on T1, with marked enhancement. Late active lesions are hypointense on T1, with variable enhancement. Inactive demyelinated, as well as early or late remyelinated lesions, will vary in T1 signal and in enhancement. Lesions show gradations in hypointensity, ranging from intense black to various shades of gray. A formal T1 hypointense lesion load can be calculated. Although chronic hypointense lesions reflect severe tissue damage, acute hypointense lesions which subsequently clear are also noted and probably reflect reversible edema/inflammation changes.

The T1 sequence is also used post contrast to evaluate enhancing lesions (Figure 6.3). Enhancement depends on contrast dose, time

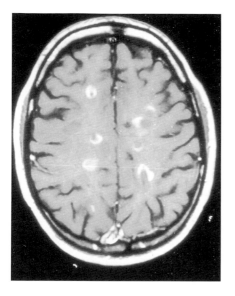

Figure 6.3
Contrast brain MRI showing multiple gadoiinium enhancing lesions.

between injection and imaging, and degree of barrier disruption. Contrast enhancement should be judged at least 5 minutes after intravenous injection of Gd-DTPA, a T1 shortening agent. If there is obvious opening of the blood–brain barrier, contrast will leak through and be visualized as a white spot on T1 imaging. Brain structures which normally enhance are the dural sinuses, cavernous sinuses, choroid plexus, infundibulum, nasopharyngeal mucosa, and pituitary gland. Gd-DTPA is given at a standard dose of 0.1 mmol/kg, but is sometimes used at double (0.2 mmol/kg) or even triple dose (0.3 mmol/kg). High dose Gd-HP-DO3A at 0.3 mmol/kg detects 47% more lesions, especially small and infratentorial lesions.[7] Contrast enhancement due to focal blood–brain barrier breakdown is associated with active lesions usually 6 weeks or less in age. The size and pattern of enhancement can be helpful. Newly visualized lesions tend to be small and intermediate in size, while previously visualized enhancing lesions appear larger. Nodular enhancement is more common with new lesions, while ring enhancement is more common with old or reactivated lesions. Although contrast lesions by definition are active, most are asymptomatic.

Contrast lesion activity is in part related to age. Young patients show the highest rates, which decrease over time. Contrast lesion activity is higher in patients with a shorter disease duration, and in relapsing vs. progressive patients. There may be seasonal fluctuation, with increased lesions in spring and early summer.[8] Use of double dose and particularly triple dose, with delayed scanning, can increase the number of detected lesions by as high as 80–120% (Figure 6.4).[9,10] The negative aspects of triple dose include increased rate of false positive lesions (small vessels and flow artifacts may be misinterpreted as lesions), greater expense, further scan delay, and length in time of the procedure.

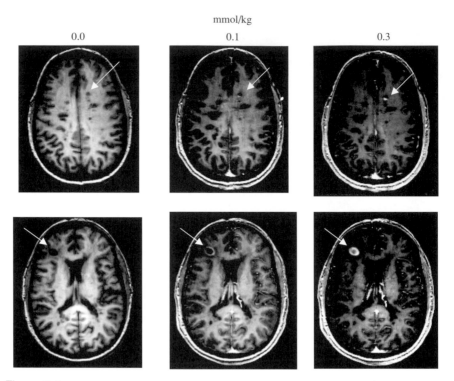

mmol/kg

0.0   0.1   0.3

Figure 6.4
Comparison of single vs. triple dose Gd-DTPA on brain MRI.

All of the above conventional sequences take some time. It can be difficult for patients to stay still, and it would be advantageous to be able to do rapid scanning. There are ways to make acquisition time much faster. Fast spin echo imaging uses multiple phase encodings in each TR, and multiple echos per TR. It allows much more rapid scanning, and thin contiguous sequences can be obtained for better signal to noise ratio. In addition, gradient echoes (echoes obtained without a 180° refocusing pulse) can be added to provide faster imaging. Echo planar speeds up data collection by use of multiechoes and multislices.

As noted earlier, T2 lesions adjacent to CSF are hard to visualize. This problem can be solved by using inversion recovery sequences, which are heavily T1W. Fluid attenuated inversion recovery (FLAIR) is an inversion recovery pulse sequence that uses a very long T1. CSF is nulled out (voided), so that it appears black (Figure 6.5). Small lesions close to CSF (cortical, juxtacortical, periventricular) are much easier to visualize,[11] and FLAIR will increase the number of detectable MS lesions. Although FLAIR requires a long acquisition time, it can be performed rapidly using fast spin echo. Another inversion recovery sequence, short tau inversion recovery (STIR), uses a very short T1 to suppress the fat signal and increase lesion detection.

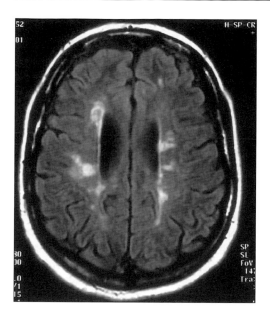

Figure 6.5
Flair sequence allows periventricular lesions to become more conspicuous because the cerebrospinal fluid appears black.

Conventional MRI techniques have major limitations. Since they detect only macroscopic changes, they have relatively low sensitivity for the true MS disease process. Lesions must be at least 2–3 mm to be visualized. Lesions that are visualized on these sequences have little pathological specificity. There is no method for distinguishing reversible from irreversible processes, particularly for T2 and PD images. It is not surprising that clinical correlation for abnormalities visualized on these conventional techniques remains limited.

Nonconventional techniques

New imaging techniques are being used in research studies and trials (Table 6.5). As they are optimized and standardized, some of these techniques are likely to become part of routine MRI analysis of MS. These nonconventional techniques offer better assessment of damage, and greater pathological specificity.

Table 6.5 New MRI techniques.

- Quantitative/volumetric measures
- Atrophy
- Magnetization transfer imaging (MTI)
- MR spectroscopy (MRS)
- Diffusion weighted imaging (DWI)
- Functional MRI (fMRI)

Role in diagnosis

MRI is the major laboratory test used to diagnose MS. At presentation brain MRI is abnormal in about 50–65% of patients, and ultimately shows lesions in 90–95% of patients. However, brain MRI loses diagnostic specificity in older subjects. After age 50 white matter lesions (most likely related to vascular changes) become more common in otherwise healthy controls. Therefore brain MRI is not as reliable a diagnostic test in older individuals.

Brain MRI used in isolation to diagnose MS can result in misdiagnosis. Without a suggestive history or examination, the incidental finding of lesions in someone being scanned to evaluate headache or head trauma has little significance for MS. Up to 4% of healthy controls will have periventricular lesions, and nonspecific white matter changes increase with age. Many disorders can produce lesions on brain MRI. However, certain features increase the likelihood that an abnormal MRI is due to MS (Table 6.8).[32–34]

The typical MS brain MRI shows T2 hyperintense lesions which are multiple, rounded, or ovoid, and which include lesions with a radial orientation

Table 6.8 Brain MRI lesion features which suggest MS.

- Number of lesions
    ≥ 4
- Size of lesions
    >3 mm diameter (esp. > 6 mm)
- Location of lesions
    - Predominantly white matter
    - Asymmetric
    - Corpus callosum involvement (sagittal T2W, lesion pointing away, moth eaten changes, atrophy)
    - Periventricular (esp. trigone and bodies, occipital/frontal lobes, floor of 4th ventricle)
    - Brainstem/infratentorial lesions
    - Juxtacortical lesions
- Shape of lesion
    - Ovoid and perpendicular to ventricle
- Contrast lesions
    - One or more contrast lesions
    - Open ring enhancement

Table 6.9 Indications for spinal MRI in the diagnosis of MS.

- Age ≥ 50 years
- Spinal cord presentation
- Normal/atypical brain MRI

to the ventricles. On T1 lesions appear hypointense. T2 lesions are always more prominent than and outnumber T1 lesions. Most new lesions enhance for 4–6 weeks. Initial enhancement involves a solid bright center, then a hyperintense ring. Open ring enhancement is said to be much more common in MS than in CNS tumor or infection.[35]

Except in special circumstances, spinal MRI is not routinely used to diagnose MS (Table 6.9). Although spinal MRI shows about 10% of the lesions noted on brain MRI, ultimately it is abnormal in 75% of patients. Using double or triple dose contrast increases the yield for lesion pickup. In a minority of MS patients (approximately 8–20%) MRI lesions may be confined to the spinal cord, with few or no brain lesions. Therefore the cord

Table 6.10 Spinal MRI lesion features which suggest MS.

- Size of lesions
  - ≤ 2 vertebral body segments in length
  - ≤ 50% of cross sectional cord area (≤15 mm)
- Location of lesion
  - Cervical (mid cervical)
  - Thoracic
  - Peripheral
- Lesions are asymmetric, multiple, scattered
- Lateral/dorsal > anterior location
- Edema only with acute lesions (often enhancing)
- Focal or diffuse atrophy

Table 6.11 Proposed diagnostic MRI criteria to demonstrate dissemination in space.[a]

Must meet three of four criteria:
1. One contrast enhancing lesion, or nine T2 hyperintense lesions
2. At least one infratentorial lesion
3. At least one juxtacortical lesion
4. At least three periventricular lesions

[a]Lesions ordinarily > 3 mm; a spinal cord lesion may substitute for a brain lesion.

Table 6.12 Proposed MRI criteria for the diagnosis of primary progressive MS.[37]

Must meet one of the following:
- At least nine T2W hyperintense lesions
- At least two spinal cord lesions
- Four to eight brain lesions plus 1 spinal cord lesion
- Four to eight brain lesions plus abnormal visual evoked potentials (VEP)
- Fewer than four brain lesions plus one spinal cord lesion plus abnormal VEP

should be imaged in patients being evaluated for MS who have normal brain MRI. There are no age-related intramedullary lesions on spinal MRI. Although spinal cord MRI is more specific, it is clearly not as sensitive as brain imaging. Certain suggestive features increase the probability that spinal MRI lesions are due to MS (Table 6.10). It is technically more difficult to image spinal cord, but recent advances include large field of view receiver coils, motion suppression, cardiac gating, and use of saturation bands.

The recent International Panel Diagnostic Guidelines rely heavily on MRI.[36] They propose specific MRI criteria to document dissemination of lesions in space, based on studies by Barkhof and Tintoré (Table 6.11),[34,35] and specific MRI criteria to make a definite diagnosis of primary progressive MS (Table 6.12).[37] Their recommended criteria to show MRI dissemination in time have been reviewed previously (see Chapter 4). It is not yet clear whether these proposed diagnostic criteria and their MRI requirements will be adopted for routine clinical use.

Recently, a Work Group on standardized MRI protocol, sponsored by the Consortium of MS Centers, has proposed a standardized brain and spinal cord protocol to use in MS (Table 6.13). These recommendations provide a starting point that will hopefully lead to a uniform application of MRI to study MS. The Work Group also proposed a common radiology report, to include a description of the findings, comparison with earlier scans, interpretation and differential diagnosis, and optimal quantitative brain volume/atrophy measures and reporting table.[38]

Table 6.13 Proposed standardized MRI protocol for MS.[38]

- Basic parameters
  - ≥ 1.0 T MRI
  - ≤ 3 mm slice thickness (≤ 1.5 mm for 3D sequences)
  - No gap
  - In plane pixel size ≤ 1 mm × 1 mm
  - Axial FSE PD/T2 : TE1 minimum < 30 ms and TE > 80 ms
  - Subcallosal line correlation for brain using three planes localizer
  - Phase array coil for spinal cord

- Brain MRI
  - Sagittal FLAIR
  - Axial FSE PD/T2, FLAIR
  - Post Gd+ (0.1 mmol/kg, 5 min delay)
  - Optional: high contrast T1 3D sequence

- Spinal Cord MRI
  - Sagittal FSE PD/T2 and T1
  - Axial FSE T2 through suspicious lesions
  - Post Gd+ (0.1–0.3 mmol/kg) sagittal SE T1 and axial SE T1 through suspicious lesions
  - Optional: high contrast T1 3D sequence

Natural history/disease pathogenesis

MRI studies have provided new insights into MS. First, serial MRI scanning indicates that the disease process is active and ongoing in most individuals despite clinical stability.[39,40] Brain lesions form in waves of activity. The 80–90% that are clinically silent are not associated with obvious relapses, or with detectable changes on the neurological examination. This ongoing lesion formation is reflected by the brain total lesion burden, which increases in untreated MS populations on average by 5–10% each year. Lesions in noneloquent areas of the brain are probably not truly silent, and are likely to contribute to eventual cognitive loss. Second, neuroimaging studies document detectable organ damage and CNS atrophy even in early and mildly affected patients.[41] MRI studies have emphasized the importance of axon involvement in this disease. Both T1 hypointense lesions and low MTR correlate with loss of axon density, and are leading to novel therapeutic strategies. Third, a number of imaging techniques show abnormalities in normal appearing CNS tissue (Table 6.14). Focal inflammation can result in distant axon injury.[42] It is clear that conventional MRI significantly underestimates the MS disease process. With techniques such as MTI and DWI focal abnormalities are reported up to 24 months before the development of conventional contrast or T2 lesions.[30] Studies have also suggested that MS may involve a diffuse but low level increase in blood–brain barrier permeability. If true, then the endothelial cell and blood–brain barrier may turn out to be key components of this disease. Fourth, MRI studies suggest that the nature of the disease process may change over time. In early stages MS is characterized by contrast lesion activity, inflammation, and relapses. Contrast lesion activity is most marked in young relapsing patients, who can show a wide range in monthly lesion number. Over time contrast lesion activity diminishes, and ultimately becomes rare. At the same time axon loss and atrophy become more prominent. This coincides roughly with the transition from relapsing to secondary progressive disease, where superimposed relapses become less and less common. MS may start out as an inflammatory and relapsing disease, only to evolve into a neurodegenerative and progressive disease.

Table 6.14 Neuroimaging techniques which detect abnormalities in normal appearing white matter/brain tissue in MS.

- MR spectroscopy
  - ↓ NAA
- Magnetization transfer imaging
  - ↓ MTR
- Diffusion weighted imaging
- Diffusion tensor imaging
- High field (esp. ≥ 4 T) MRI

Fifth, MRI has provided insights into lesion heterogeneity. Some are more destructive than others. Not all hyperintense T2/PD lesions are hypointense on T1, consistent with more severe tissue damage. Lesions show variable MTR changes.[17] T1 hypointense lesions have lower MTR than isointense lesions. Lesions which are only detected on triple dose Gd-DPTA have a higher MTR value than lesions which enhance on single dose.[43] Homogeneously enhancing lesions have higher MTR than ring enhancing lesions, consistent with the notion that they are new rather than old reactivated lesions. Lesions which enhance on at least two monthly scans have lower MTR values than lesions which enhance on a single scan, suggesting prolonged enhancement is associated with more severe tissue damage. Longitudinal lesion assessment, using MTR, indicates marked heterogeneity in lesion recovery. Only a minority of lesions (5–13%) in early relapsing MS patients showed continued decrease in MTR over several months. Secondary progressive patients show lower MTR values for new lesions than relapsing patients, consistent with more severe pathological damage. Sixth, studies suggest that tissue changes and demyelination can occur independent of focal blood–brain barrier impairment.[30,44] Finally, MRI finds group differences between MS clinical subtypes including benign, relapsing, secondary progressive, and primary progressive MS (Table 6.15). With conventional techniques, secondary progressive patients have more T1 hypointense lesions, ventricular enlargement, and spinal cord atrophy.[45] Primary progressive patients have more diffuse brain and spinal cord abnormalities.[46] With regard to whole brain MTR histograms, relapsing patients show lower MTR histogram image peak heights than benign relapsing patients. Secondary progressive patients show lower NAA in normal appearing white matter than relapsing patients.[47] Secondary progressive MS patients have the lowest MTR histogram measurements,[48] while primary progressive patients have lower peak heights, normal peak position, and overall relatively normal histograms. The primary progressive MTR findings suggest a subtle but diffuse change even within normal appearing white matter. Although it is not possible with current imaging to determine MS subtype, group differences are important clues to better understand the pathogenesis of MS. Progressive MS subtypes have greater MTR changes in the cervical cord than relapsing patients.[49] Classic primary progressive MS is associated with more obvious spinal cord disease, relatively little contrast lesion activity and accumulating burden of disease, marked atrophy, and diffuse disturbances in normal appearing CNS tissue.[47] The fact that T2 lesions are more likely to be hypointense on T1 in secondary progressive vs. relapsing patients suggests a failure of recovery or repair mechanisms, or the occurrence of more destructive lesions.

Table 6.15 Neuroimaging differences between MS clinical subtypes.

Subtype	MR features
Primary progressive	Low brain lesion burden Low contrast lesion activity More pronounced spinal cord changes (including atrophy) Diffuse brain and spinal cord abnormalities Normal brain MTR histogram (↓ peak heights)
Benign relapsing	Normal lesion NAA ↓↓ T2 lesion load ↓↓ T1 hypointense lesions ↑ Brain MTR histogram Low contrast lesion activity
Relapsing	↓ T2 lesion load ↓ T1 hypointense lesions ↑ MTR in new lesions ↓ Brain MTR histogram
Secondary progressive	Most marked CNS atrophy More confluent cerebral and cerebellum lesions More periventricular, brainstem lesions ↑ T1 hypointense lesions ↓ Cerebral lesions ↓ MTR in new lesions ↓↓ Brain MTR histogram Most marked abnormalities in normal appearing CNS tissue ↓ NAA ↓ MTR

Role in prognosis/correlative features

Conventional MRI markers are most predictive of future disease course in first attack patients. These patients have no prior neurological history. They present with either a clinically isolated syndrome (CIS), such as unilateral optic neuritis, incomplete transverse myelitis, or isolated brainstem/cerebellar syndrome picture, or a multifocal clinical syndrome. Approximately 65% of such patients show multifocal brain MRI lesions. Under the age of 50, unexplained T2 lesions predict development of clinically definite MS. Of first attack patients with abnormal brain MRI, 30% will develop clinically definite MS within 1 year,[50] 50% by 5 years,[51] 80% by 10 years,[52] and 88% by 14 years.[53] By contrast, only 19% of patients with normal brain MRI and unifocal clinical presentation develop MS during a 14-year follow-up. Risk is higher with a multifocal clinical presentation.[54] The presence of contrast lesions on the baseline MRI increases risk of early conversion to MS (within 3 years), as does number and volume of T2 lesions (within 5 years). Lesion number and size predicts at 10 years not only MS subtype (benign, relapsing, or secondary progressive), but also disability (as measured by EDSS). In a prospective study of 81 CIS patients, 83% with abnormal brain MRI had developed clinically definite MS by 10 years.[52] Of those, 39% had mild relapsing MS, 20% had relapsing MS, and 24% had secondary progressive MS. By contrast, of CIS patients with normal brain MRI only 11% had MS, and all had mild disease. In this series initial brain lesion number correlated with EDSS and clinical subtype at 10 years, but the association between EDSS and lesion number and volume was strongest in the first 5 years. Over the first 5 years after presentation, brain lesion load increased the least for mild MS, was intermediate for relapsing MS, and was greatest for secondary progressive MS. Those with a lesion volume greater than 3 cm^3 had a 100% conversion to MS within 4 years, and 45% had an EDSS greater than 6 at 10 years.[55] Of those with a lesion volume of less than 3 cm^3, 78% had developed MS within less than 7 years but only 18% had an EDSS greater than 6. In this same cohort, 71 patients were followed for 14 years. A second clinical attack developed in 88% of those with an abnormal MRI presentation, compared to 19% of those with a normal MRI. However, further clinical or MRI activity occurred in 98% of those with abnormal MRI at presentation compared to 38% of those with a normal MRI.[53] The strongest correlation with ultimate disability was the number and size of lesions on the first scan, and the increase in lesion volume in the first 5 years. In summary, in CIS patients initial MRI seems to predict the long term risk of MS, the MS clinical subtype, and the degree of disability.

For established MS patients, a number of MRI features have been said to have prognostic significance (Table 6.16).[56] Conventional MRI markers (T2

Table 6.16 MRI features with prognostic significance.

- Atrophy
  - ↑ Brain atrophy
  - ↑ Spinal cord atrophy

- Hypointense T1W lesions
  - ↑ T1 lesion load

- MTR changes
  - ↓ MTR histogram

- Total lesion burden
  - ↑ T2 lesion load

- Number and volume of enhancing lesions
  - ↑ Contrast lesions

- Number and volume of active lesions
  - ↑ New, enlarging, contrast lesions

- MR spectroscopy changes
  - ↓ NAA

lesion load and contrast activity) are not as strongly predictive of future course as in first attack patients. Nonconventional markers appear more promising in this regard. Contrast lesion activity does show good correlation with relapses, clinical symptoms, T2 lesion burden, and subsequent enhancing lesions. It shows less correlation with atrophy, disability, and disease progression. In relapsing patients contrast lesion activity is associated with increased relapse rate over the next year,[57] and relapses are more likely to occur in patients who show enhancing lesions. Activity on 6-monthly scans has greater predictive value than activity on a single scan.[58] Contrast lesion activity and T2 lesion load are weakly predictive for future disability in relapsing MS,[58,59] and these conventional markers show even less predictive value for disability in secondary progressive MS. Chronic hypointense lesions, which indicate more tissue destruction, show better prognostic significance. T1 lesion load is a better disability correlate than T2 lesion load, and increase in T1 lesion load correlates with increase in disability.[60-62]

CNS atrophy is one of the most promising MRI markers of disability. Spinal cord atrophy, as measured by mean cord diameter at C2, correlates with both EDSS and disease duration in relapsing MS.[63] Secondary progressive patients show much smaller cord diameters than relapsing patients.[64] When measured by volumetric techniques, spinal cord atrophy correlates with continued functional status scores even more so than with EDSS.[65] Studies also suggest that increasing brain atrophy also correlates with increasing disability.[66,67] Whole brain MTR histogram is another nonconventional technique that correlates with brain atrophy, T2 lesion volume, and T1 lesion volume. It is said to show strong correlation with clinical disability. Progression

Table 6.17 MRI markers associated with cognitive loss in MS.

- Lesion load
  - ↑ T2 lesion load (esp. ≥ 30 cm³)
  - ↑ Frontal, parietal T2 lesion load
  - ↑ Hypointense T1 lesion load
  - ↑ Juxtacortical lesion burden

- Atrophy
  - Brain volume
  - Corpus callosum atrophy
  - Ventricular enlargement

- Confluent periventricular lesions

- Frontal lobe lesions (problems in conceptual reasoning)

- MTI parameters
  - ↓ MTR histogram in normal appearing brain tissue and white matter
  - ↓ Average lesion MTR

- MRS parameters
  - ↓ Periventricular NAA

of disability also correlates with decreased NAA in normal appearing white matter.[68] The relationship between decrease in NAA and increase in EDSS (disability) is stronger for relapsing than secondary progressive MS.

Among the many symptoms of MS, cognitive dysfunction is one of the most bothersome. A number of studies have reported MRI abnormalities associated with cognitive dysfunction (Table 6.17).

Outcome measure in clinical trials

MRI is routinely used as an outcome measure in clinical trials to assess both acute and chronic disease changes (Table 6.18).[69,70] Active lesions can be new, enlarging, or enhancing, and total lesion volume can be calculated to give the burden of disease/total lesion load. A task force of the National MS Society suggested in 1996 that MRI (serial monthly T2 and contrast brain studies) could be used as a primary outcome measure in exploratory studies of new treatments.[71] However, they recommended that MRI remain a secondary outcome measure in definitive phase III trials of relapsing and secondary progressive MS. Preliminary trials typically last for 6–12 months, while definitive trials are conducted for 2–3 years. MRI is typically done monthly in preliminary trials, and at 6–12 months in definitive trials. The Task Force suggested that MRI could be used to select appropriate first attack patients for therapeutic trials to prevent conversion to definite MS. This was done for the CHAMPS and ETOMS studies. A recent workshop emphasized that conventional MRI remains an unvalidated MS surrogate.[72] Although MRI clearly reflects disease pathobiology, no single measure is sufficient to capture the disease process, and multiple measures should be used. The workshop emphasized that in trials for which MRI is the primary outcome, an extension phase is important to document drug

Table 6.18 MRI as an outcome measure in clinical trials.

- Acute disease changes
  - Number of contrast lesions
  - Contrast lesion load

- Chronic disease changes
  - Number of T2 lesions
  - T2 lesion load
  - T1 hypointense lesion load

- Combined changes
  - Combined unique (T2 and T1Gd+) lesions

- In relation to patient groups
  - Proportion of active scans per patient
  - Proportion of patients with/without active scans/lesions

effects and safety over a longer period of time. Drug mechanism of action must be considered, since a novel drug might be beneficial yet not affect MRI. Treatments may also have MRI effects that are not the result of change in the predicted disease pathology.

There are several suggested trial designs for exploratory therapeutic studies (Figure 6.7). Using frequent MRI scans, they allow studies to be done on relatively small numbers of patients. Monthly MRI scans, performed over 6 months in a parallel group design, require about 40 relapsing patients in each arm to show a 60% reduction in new enhancing lesions.[73] Performing a 1-month run-in scan further reduces the required sample size by 30%.[74] Crossover designs take advantage of the fact that

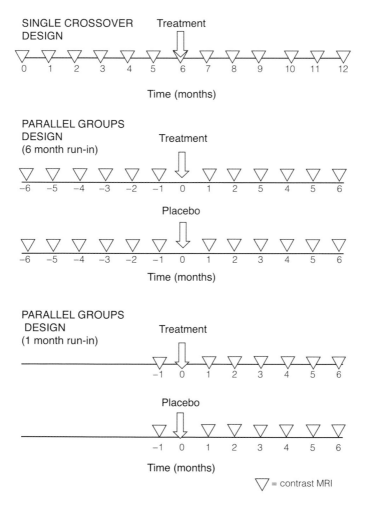

Figure 6.7
Recommended trial design for phase II/exploratory studies.

Table 6.19 Recommended MRI outcomes for MS therapeutic trials.[78]

	CIS	Relapsing	Secondary progressive	Primary progressive
Primary outcome	T2 lesion load Contrast lesions	T2 lesion load Contrast lesions	T2 lesion load Contrast lesions Brain volume T1 hypointense lesion load	T2 lesion load Contrast lesions Brain volume T1 hypointense lesion load
Secondary outcome	Brain volume T1 hypointense lesion load	Brain volume T1 hypointense lesion load	MTR histogram Spinal cord volume MRS	MTR histogram Spinal cord volume MRS
Tertiary outcome	–	–	Diffusion parameters T2 decay analysis T1 relaxation time	Diffusion parameters T2 decay analysis T1 relaxation time

there is less intrapatient variability to lower required numbers even further. Using a 6-month run-in, and 6 months on treatment, 10–12 patients can be used to show a 60% reduction in activity. These estimates are based largely on relapsing patients, and secondary progressive trials probably require larger numbers of patients.[27,75,76]. About 67% of relapsing or secondary progressive patients will develop contrast lesions during a 3-month observation period.

In definitive phase III treatment trials, MRI provides confirmatory evidence for treatment effect. It also provides important insight into the disease process which can lead to new information about MS. T2 imaging allows calculation of lesion burden, as well as new or enlarging lesions. At the least this should be done at the beginning and end of the study, but more often is done every 6–12 months. Two run-in and two exit scans can help to compensate for monthly MRI variations.[27] Rather than all the patients in a study undergoing contrast MRI, it can be reserved for a subgroup at selected trial centers, and done monthly for 6 months at the beginning and end of the trial. Recent recommendations suggest the addition of measures such as atrophy, T1 hypointense lesions, MRS, MTI, and DWI to phase III trials to improve specificity of changes (Table 6.19). Nonconventional MRI measures will become more important in future clinical trials.

Trials typically use a central MRI reading group, require that study sites be able to obtain adequate images, and require standardized protocols (including sequences and positioning).[77] In analyzing MRI trial data, subgroup analysis based on the baseline T2 lesion load or presence of contrast lesions may be useful.

MRI effects are always more marked than clinical effects in treatment trials. In most cases, clinical and MRI outcome results are consistent. However, there are examples in secondary progressive MS patients where a treatment was able to shut down contrast lesion formation and stabilize T2 burden of disease, yet patients continued to progress with ongoing atrophy and clinical disability. The most likely explanation for this clinical–MRI discrepancy is the occurrence of ongoing axon loss despite control of inflammation and edema. It is consistent with the current belief that disease progression in the later phases of MS reflects a neurodegenerative process rather than an inflammatory one.

Current role

MRI is being used in MS in four different ways (Table 6.20). First, it is an integral part of the diagnostic workup. In most cases this is brain MRI with contrast, but spinal cord MRI is indicated for diagnosis in selected cases. If it is done with contrast, double or even triple dose should be considered. Second, MRI is included in virtually all MS therapeutic trials. In most cases both T2 and contrast lesion activity, as well as T2 lesion burden, are meas-

Table 6.20 Current use of MRI in MS.

- As part of the diagnostic workup
  - Brain MRI with contrast
  - Spinal cord MRI with double/triple dose contrast (in selected cases)

- As a surrogate outcome measure in therapeutic trials
  - Most appropriate for relapsing and secondary progressive MS
  - Primary outcome in phase II/exploratory clinical trials
  - Secondary/tertiary outcomes in phase III/pivotal trials

- As a disease activity marker
  - To assess pretreatment baseline/disease severity
  - To monitor response to therapy

- As a research tool
  - To study extent of CNS abnormalities
  - To determine the nature of CNS involvement

ured. Third, MRI remains the best laboratory marker of disease activity. It is used increasingly by clinicians to help guide choice of disease-modifying therapy, to provide a pretreatment baseline assessment, and to monitor whether a patient is a suboptimal or nonresponder to disease-modifying therapy. It provides objective evidence of disease-related damage. Finally, MRI is being used in research studies to learn more about the nature and extent of CNS injury.

Future role

In the future, the role of MRI in MS is likely to expand. Developments will occur in several areas. First, there is increasing pressure to develop standardized protocols for diagnostic use of MRI in MS. This would involve specified sequences, slice thickness, positioning, and dosing (timing of contrast), so that the quality as well as comparability of scans is enhanced. There is also increasing pressure to develop accepted MRI criteria for diagnosis at the time of first attack. Second, nonconventional MRI techniques are being standardized and evaluated to examine whether they can be extended to routine clinical use. Computerized programs to measure T2/T1 lesion burden, contrast lesion burden, atrophy, and whole brain NAA are likely to be widely available in the next few years. These improved surrogate outcome markers are likely to be routinely assessed in clinical trials, perhaps allowing smaller numbers of patients to be used. Third, consensus guidelines are needed to standardize and guide how MRI should be used to follow response to disease-modifying therapy. Finally, MRI is being applied to new research areas. It is possible to use MRI to track movement of single cell populations. This could provide insight not only into how cells get into the CNS in MS, but also what happens to them when they get there. MRI techniques which measure specific pathological processes, such as demyelination, remyelination, and axon damage, are needed to assess disease severity and response to treatment. MS appears to be a heterogeneous disorder. Distinct immunopathological patterns are described, and MRI correlates are being sought. In the future MRI may be used to help determine pathologically heterogeneous groups of patients.

References

1. Khoury SJ, Weiner HL. Multiple sclerosis. What have we learned from magnetic resonance imaging studies? Arch Intern Med 1998; 158:565–573.

2. Miller DH. Guidelines for MRI monitoring of the treatment of multiple sclerosis: recommendations of the US Multiple Sclerosis Society's task force. Mult Scler 1996; 1:335–338.

3. Schwartz GM, Huang Y. Relating frequency to space: the Fourier transform. In: Woodward P, ed. MRI for technologists, 2nd edn. New York: McGraw-Hill; 2001:39–54.

4. Brex PA, Parker GJM, Leary SM, et al. Lesion heterogeneity in multiple sclerosis: a study of the relations between appearances on T1 weighted images, T1 relaxation times, and metabolite concentrations. J Neurol Neurosurg Psychiatry 2000; 68:627–632.

5. Van Walderveen MA, Kamphorst W, Scheltens P, et al. Histopathological correlate of hypointense lesions on T1-weighted spin-echo MRI in multiple sclerosis. Neurology 1998,50:1282–1288.

6. Van Walderveen MA, Lycklama A, Nijeholt GJ, Ader HJ, et al. Hypointense lesions on T1-weighted spin-echo magnetic resonance imaging. Arch Neurology 2001; 58:76–81.

7. Koudriavtseva T, Pozzilli C, DiBiasi C, et al. High-dose contrast-enhanced MRI in multiple sclero-sis. Neuroradiology 1996; 38:S5–S9.

8. Auer DP, Schumann EM, Kümpfel T, et al. Seasonal fluctuations of gadolinium-enhancing magnetic resonance imaging lesions in multiple sclerosis. Ann Neurol 2000; 47:276–277.

9. Filippi M, Capra R, Campi A, et al. Triple dose of gadolinium-DTPA and delayed MRI in patients with benign multiple sclerosis. J Neurol Neurosurg Psychiatry 1996; 60:526–530.

10. Silver NC, Good GJ, Barker GJ, et al. Sensitivity of contrast enhanced MRI in multiple sclerosis. Effects of gadolinium dose, magnetization transfer contrast and delayed imaging. Brain 1997; 120:1149–1161.

11. Miller DH, Grossman RI, Reingold SC and McFarland HF. The role of magnetic resonance techniques in understanding and managing multiple sclerosis. BRAIN 1998; 121:3–24.

12. Pfefferbaum A, Mathalon DH, Sullivan EV, et al. A quantitative magnetic resonance imaging study of changes in brain morphology from infancy to late adulthood. Arch Neurol 1994; 51:874–887.

13. Gur RC, Mozley PD, Resnick SM, et al. Gender differences in age effect on brain atrophy measured by magnetic resonance imaging. Proc Natl Acad Sci USA 1991; 88:2845–2849.

14. Paolillo A, Pozzilli C, Gasperini C, et al. Brain atrophy in relapsing-

remitting multiple sclerosis: relationship with "black holes", disease duration and clinical disability. J Neurol Sci 2000; 174:85–91.

15. Dousset V, Gayou A, Brochet B, et al. Early structural changes in acute MS lesions assessed by serial magnetization transfer studies. Neurology 1998; 51:1150–1155.

16. Filippi M. In-vivo tissue characterization of multiple sclerosis and other white matter diseases using magnetic resonance based techniques. J. Neurol. 2001; 248:1019–1029.

17. Filippi M, Rocca MA, Minicucci L, et al. Magnetization transfer imaging of patients with definite MS and negative conventional MRI. Neurology1999; 52:845–848.

18. Tortorella C, Viti B, Bozzali M, et al. A magnetization transfer histogram study of normal appearing brain tissue in MS. Neurology 2000; 54:186–193.

19. Bozzali M, Rocca MA, Iannucci G, et al. Magnetization-transfer histogram analysis of the cervical cord in patients with multiple sclerosis. Am J Neuroradiol 1999; 20:1803–1808.

20. Simon JH, Jacobs LD, Campion MK, et al. A longitudinal study of brain atrophy in relapsing multiple sclerosis. Neurology 1999; 53:139–148.

21. Bitsch A, Bruhn H, Vougioukas, et al. Inflammatory CNS demyelination: histopathological correlation with in vivo quantitative proton MR spectroscopy. Am J Neuroradiol 1999; 20:1619–1627.

22. Gonen O, Catalaa I, Babb JS, et al. Total brain N-acetylaspartate. A new measure of disease load in MS. Neurology 2000; 54:15–19.

23. Leary SM, Davie CA, Parker GJM, et al. ¹H magnetic resonance spectroscopy of normal appearing white matter in primary progressive multiple sclerosis. J Neurol 1999; 246:1023–1026.

24. Sarchielli P, Presciutti O, Pelliccioli P, et al. Absolute quantification of brain metabolites by proton magnetic resonance spectroscopy in normal-appearing white matter of multiple sclerosis patients. Brain 1999; 122:513–521.

25. De Stefano N, Matthews PM, Antel PJ, et al. Chemical pathology of acute demyelinating lesions and its correlation with disability. Ann Neurol 1995; 38:901–909.

26. Cucurella M-G, Rovira A, Rio J, et al. Proton magnetic resonance spectroscopy in primary and secondary progressive multiple sclerosis. NMR Biomed 2000; 13:57–63.

27. Miller DH, Grossman RI, Reingold SC, McFarland HF. The role of magnetic resonance techniques in understanding and managing multiple sclerosis. Brain 1998; 121:3–24.

28. Cercignani M, Iannucci G, Filippi M. Diffusion-weighted imaging in multiple sclerosis. Ital J. Neurol Sci 1999; 20:S246–S249.

29. Nusbaum AO, Tang CY, Wei T-C, et al. Whole-brain diffusion MR histograms differ between MS subtypes. Neurology 2000; 54:1421–1426.

30. Werring DJ, Brassat D, Droogan G, et al. The pathogenesis of lesions and normal-appearing white matter changes in multiple sclerosis. A serial diffusion MRI study. Brain 2000; 123:1667–1676.

31. Lee M, Reddy H, Johansen-Berg H, et al. The motor cortex shows adaptive functional changes to brain injury from multiple sclerosis. Ann Neurol 2000; 47:606–613.

32. Fazekas F, Barkhof F, Filippi M. Unenhanced and enhanced magnetic resonance imaging in the

diagnosis of multiple sclerosis. J Neurol Neurosurg Psychiatry 1998; 64:S2–S5.

33. Barkhof F, Filippi M, Miller DH, et al. Comparison of MRI criteria at first presentation to predict conversion to clinically definite multiple sclerosis. Brain 1997; 120:2059–2069.

34. Tintoré M, Rovira A, Martinez M, Rio J, et al. Isolated demyelinating syndromes: comparison of different MR imaging criteria to predict conversion to clinically definite multiple sclerosis. Am J Neuroradiol 2000; 21:702–706.

35. Masdeu JC, Quinto C, Olivera C, et al. Open-ring imaging sign. Highly specific for atypical brain demyelination. Neurology 2000; 54:1427–1423.

36. McDonald WI, Compston A, Edan G, et al. Recommended diagnostic criteria for multiple sclerosis: guidelines from the International Panel on the diagnosis of multiple sclerosis. Ann Neurol 2001; 50:121–127.

37. Thompson AJ, Montalban X, Barkoff et al. Diagnostic criteria for primary progressive multiple sclerosis: a position paper. Ann Neurol 2000; 47: 831–835.

38. Traboulsee T. ENS 2002 Guidelines for a standardized MRI Protocal for MS. CMSC Professional Forum. http://www.mscare.org/forums/ viewtopic.php?+=36

39. Simone IL, Tortorella C, Federico F. The contribution of ^{1}H-magnetic resonance spectroscopy in defining the pathophysiology of multiple sclerosis. Ital J Neurol Sci 1999; 20:S241–S245.

40. Stone LA, Frank JA, Albert PA, et al. The effect of interferon β on blood–brain barrier disruptions demonstratable by contrast-enhanced MRI in relapsing remitting MS. Ann Neurol 1995; 37:611–619.

41. Rudick RA, Fisher E, Lee J-C, et al. Use of the brain parenchymal fraction to measure whole brain atrophy in relapsing-remitting MS. Neurology 1999; 53:1698–1704.

42. Simon JH, Kinkel RP, Jacobs L, et al. A Wallerian degeneration pattern in patients at risk for MS. Neurology 2000; 54:1155–1160.

43. Filippi M, Rocca MA, Rizzo G, et al. Magnetization transfer ratios in multiple sclerosis lesions enhancing after different doses of gadolinium. Neurology 1998; 50:1289–1293.

44. Narayana PA, Doyle TJ, Lai D, Wolinsky JS. Serial proton magnetic resonance spectroscopic imaging, contrast-enhanced magnetic resonance imaging, and quantitative lesion volumetry in multiple sclerosis. Ann Neurol 1998; 43:56–71.

45. Nijeholt GJ, van Walderveen MA, Castelijns JA, et al. Brain and spinal cord abnormalities in multiple sclerosis. Correlation between MRI parameters, clinical subtypes and symptoms. Brain 1998; 121:687–697.

46. Lycklama à Nijeholt GJ, Van Walderveen MA, Castelijns JA, et al. Brain and spinal cord abnormalities in multiple sclerosis. Brain 1998; 121:687–697.

47. Tourbah A, Stievenart JL, Gout O, et al. Localized proton magnetic resonance spectroscopy in relapsing remitting versus secondary progressive multiple sclerosis. Neurology 1999; 53:1091–1097.

48. Rovaris M, Bozzali M, Santiccio G, et al. Relative contributions of brain and cervical cord pathology to multiple sclerosis disability: a study with magnetization transfer ration histogram analysis. J Neurol Neurosurg Psychiatry 2000; 69:723–727.

49. Filippi M, Bozzali M, Horsfield MA, et al. A conventional and magneti-

zation transfer MRI study of the cervical cord in patients with MS. Neurology 2000; 54:207–213.

50. Brex PA, O'Riordan JI, Miszkiel KA, et al. Multisequence MRI in clinically isolated syndromes and the early development of MS. Neurology 1999; 53:1184–1190.

51. Optic Neuritis Study Group. The 5-year risk of MS after optic neuritis. Experience of the optic neuritis treatment trial. Neurology 1997; 49:1404–1413.

52. O'Riordan JI, Thompson AJ, Kingsley DP, et al. The prognostic value of brain MRI in clinically isolated syndromes of the CNS. A 10-year follow-up. Brain 1998; 121:495–503.

53. Brex PA, Ciccarelli O, O'Riordan JI, et al. A longitudinal study of abnormalities on MRI and disability from multiple sclerosis. N Engl J Med 2002; 346:158–164.

54. Comi G, Filippi M, Barkhoff F, et al. Effect of early interferon treatment on conversion to definite multiple sclerosis: a randomised study. Lancet 2001; 357:1576–1582.

55. Sailer M, O'Riordan JI, Thompson AJ, et al. Quantitative MRI in patients with clinically isolated syndromes suggestive of demyelination. Neurology 1999; 52:599–606.

56. Weiner HL, Guttman CRG, Khoury SJ, et al. Serial magnetic resonance imaging in multiple sclerosis: correlation with attacks, disability, and disease stage. J Neuroimmunol 2000; 104:164–173.

57. Molyneux PD, Filippi M, Barkhof F et al. Correlations between monthly enhanced MRI lesion rate and changes in T2 lesion volume in multiple sclerosis. Ann Neurol 1998; 43:332–339.

58. Kappos L, Moeri D, Radue EW, et al. Predictive value of gadolinium-enhanced magnetic resonance imaging for relapse rate and changes in disability or impairment in multiple sclerosis: a meta-analysis. Lancet 1999; 353:964–969.

59. Filippi M, Paty DW, Kappos L, et al. Correlations between changes in disability and T2-weighted brain MRI activity in multiple sclerosis: a follow-up study. Neurology 1995; 45:255–260.

60. Truyen L, Van Waesberghe, Van Walderveen MAA, et al. Accumulation of hypointense lesions ("black holes") on T1 spin-echo MRI correlates with disease progression in multiple sclerosis. Neurology 1996; 47:1469–1476.

61. Van Waesberghe JHTM, Kamphorst W, De Groot CJA, et al. Axonal loss in multiple sclerosis lesions: magnetic resonance imaging insights into substrates of disability. Ann Neurol 1999; 46:747–754.

62. Van Walderveen MA, Barkhof F, Hommes OR, et al. Correlating MRI and clinical disease activity in multiple sclerosis: relevance of hypointense lesion on short-TR/short-TE (T1 weighted) spin echo images. Neurology 1995; 45:1684–1690.

63. Losseff NA, Webb SL, O'Riordan JI et al. Spinal cord atrophy and disability in multiple sclerosis. A new reproducible and sensitive MRI method with potential to monitor disease progression. Brain 1996; 119:701–708.

64. Stevenson VL, Leary SM, Losseff NA, et al. Spinal cord atrophy and disability in MS: a longitudinal study. Neurology 1998; 51:234–238.

65. Fox NC, Jenkins R, Leary SM, et al. Progressive cerebral atrophy in MS. A serial study using registered, volumetric MRI. Neurology 2000; 54:807–812.

66. Ge Y, Grossman RI, Udupa JK, et al. Brain atrophy in relapsing-remitting multiple sclerosis and secondary progressive multiple

sclerosis: longitudinal quantitative analysis. Radiology 2000; 214:665–670.

67. Losseff NA, Wang L, Lai HM, et al. Progressive cerebral atrophy in multiple sclerosis. A serial MRI study. Brain 1996; 119:2009–2019.

68. Fu L, Matthews PM, De Stefano N, et al. Imaging axonal damage of normal-appearing white matter in multiple sclerosis. Brain 1998; 121:103–113.

69. Erickson BJ, Noseworthy JH. Value of magnetic resonance imaging in assessing efficacy in clinical trials of multiple sclerosis therapies. Mayo Clin Proc 1997; 72:1080–1089.

70. Evans AC, Frank JA, Antel J, Miller DH. The role of MRI in clinical trial of multiple sclerosis: comparison of image processing techniques. Ann Neurol 1997; 41:125–132.

71. Miller DH, Albert PS, Barkhoff F, et al. Guidelines for the use of magnetic resonance techniques in monitoring the treatment of multiple sclerosis. Ann Neurol 1996; 39:6–16.

72. Joy JE, Johnston Jr RB (eds). Multiple sclerosis. Current status and strategies for the future. Washington DC: National Academy Press; 2001.

73. McFarland HF, Frank JA, Albert PS, et al. Using gadolinium-enhanced magnetic resonance imaging lesions to monitor disease activity in multiple sclerosis. Ann Neurol 1992; 32:758–766.

74. Nauta JJ, Thompson AJ, Barkhoff F, Miller DH. Magnetic resonance imaging in monitoring the treatment of multiple sclerosis patients: statistical power of parallel-groups and crossover designs. J Neurol Sci 1994; 122:6–14.

75. Tubridy N, Ader HJ, Barkhoff, et al. Exploratory treatment trials in multiple sclerosis using MRI: sample size calculations for relapsing-remitting and secondary progressive subgroups using placebo controlled parallel groups. J Neurol Neurosurg Psychiatry 1998; 64:50–55.

76. Tubridy N, Ader HJ, Barkhoff, et al. Sample size calculations for MRI outcome pilot trials in multiple sclerosis: relapsing-remitting versus secondary progressive subgroups. Neurology 1997; 48:A175.

77. Tofts PS. Standardisation and optimisation of magnetic resonance techniques for multicentre studies. J Neurol Neurosurg Psychiatry 1998; 64:S37–S43.

7
Disease-modifying therapy

Treatment of acute exacerbations

The treatment of acute exacerbations of MS has centered on use of corticosteroids or ACTH. There have been few well designed, controlled studies on steroid use since the initial study of Rose in 1970.[1] In that study, patients treated with ACTH improved more rapidly than those treated with placebo. But the beneficial effect was only evident for a few weeks, with no long-term difference seen between the two groups. Subsequent studies have utilized intravenous methylprednisolone. Although none of these studies would be considered pivotal, they suggested a short-term benefit from steroid. While there are few data to recommend one form of corticosteroid over another, or an optimal dosing schedule, most centers utilize a 3- to 5-day course of methylprednisolone, intravenous, 1 gram daily, optionally followed by a short course of rapidly tapered oral prednisone. A meta-analysis of three studies comparing the effect of IV high dose steroid to placebo on recovery of expanded disability status scale (EDSS) confirmed the benefit of high dose steroid when assessed up to 28 days after treatment.[2] The same study evaluated two dose-testing regimens and could not find a short term difference between high and low dose steroids. One of the major design problems of clinical trials of therapy for acute exacerbations is that patients were entered at too long a period after onset of the acute attack. In the Rose study and others, patients were entered as long as 8 weeks after onset, a period that could allow for spontaneous recovery to obscure any treatment effect.

A recent study of an adhesion molecule blocker (see below), in which there was a placebo group and a group that received methylprednisolone, 1 g daily for 3 days, demonstrated that methylprednisolone was significantly better than placebo (or the adhesion molecule blocker) at reducing measures of disability/impairment. This effect persisted through at least 90 days. The safety of using oral steroids in moderate doses (60–100 mg/day) was a concern following the Optic Neuritis Treatment Trial, where an increased frequency of recurrent optic neuritis was seen in the oral steroid treated group. These results have not been confirmed (or refuted) by additional studies. It is not clear whether equivalent higher doses of oral steroids are as beneficial as those given IV.

The importance of treating acute exacerbations was highlighted by an analysis of the placebo groups from several of the recent clinical trials of disease-altering therapies. As the patients were followed with assessments every 3 months, one could gauge the effect of an acute attack on measures of neurological function, e.g. EDSS and Scripps score. The analysis revealed that there was a measurable worsening of both scores that was apparent within 3 months after the exacerbation and persisted through subsequent study visits. For the EDSS residual deficit was seen in 43% of exacerbations, with a mean residual worsening of 0.4 EDSS points. For the Scripps score, residual deficit was seen in 52% of patients, with a mean residual worsening of 1.6 points (Figure 7.1). These results provide compelling data that relapses are detrimental and incomplete recovery from relapses is an important cause of accrued disability. Therefore, therapies that reduce relapse rate may be beneficial, independent of their ability to affect the progressive aspect of this illness.

The use of adhesion molecule blockers was a theoretically attractive approach to treating acute exacerbations, in the hope that by blocking trafficking of lymphocytes into the CNS, one could lessen the effects of an acute attack. Two trials attempted to utilize this approach. The first employed a monoclonal antibody directed against CD11/CD18 in an attempt to block LFA1 on lymphocytes as well as adhesion molecules on macrophages and neutrophils. Patients were treated with one of two doses of the monoclonal antibody, methylprednisolone, 1 g daily for 3 days, or placebo, with provisions for a steroid rescue. Treatment had to be initiated within 7 days of the acute attack. The results did not demonstrate any effect of the adhesion blocking agent, but demonstrated that IV methylprednisolone produced a significantly better outcome than placebo (or the monoclonal antibody) that persisted through at least 90 days (Figure 7.2).

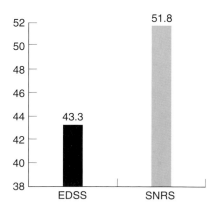

Figure 7.1
Percentage of patients with residual worsening on the EDSS and Scripps scales after an exacerbation.

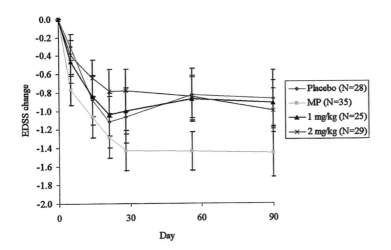

Figure 7.2
Effect of an adhesion molecule blocking agent, methylprednisolone, and placebo on recovery from an acute exacerbation of MS IV methylprednisolone provided significantly greater improvement.

The second study employed a monoclonal antibody directed against the integrin VLA-4 on lymphocytes. In animal models, blockage of this molecule produced amelioration of experimental autoimmune encephalomyelitis (EAE). In this study, patients were entered within 96 hours of the acute exacerbation. This study also failed to demonstrate a beneficial effect from blocking adhesion molecules. These results suggest that at the time that an acute exacerbation becomes clinically apparent, it is too late to attempt to block the entry of cells into the CNS. Alternately, the entire approach may be wrong. Additional studies are underway to determine if more chronic therapy with adhesion molecule blocking agents will affect the course of MS.

Disease-altering therapies

In 1993, the FDA approved the first agent for altering the course of MS, interferon β-1b, ushering in the era of disease-modifying treatments for MS. In 1996, interferon β-1a, for intramuscular use, was approved for relapsing forms of MS and later in 1996, glatiramer acetate was approved for relapsing-remitting MS (RRMS). In 1999 mitoxantrone was approved for worsening MS. A subcutaneously administered preparation of interferon β-1a was approved for use in relapsing MS in the USA in 2002, but had been available earlier in Canada and Europe.

Interferon β-1b

The first study to demonstrate the effectiveness of systemically administered interferon β was the North American Interferon β-1b (Betaseron)
study, which started in 1988.[3] This study utilized a double blind, placebo
controlled design. The inclusion criteria were patients with relapsing-
remitting disease, Kurtzke EDSS scores of 0–5.5, and two or more exacerbations in the prior 2 years. Data were obtained from 372 patients
randomized to receive placebo, 1.6 MIU interferon β, or 8 MIU interferon β,
subcutaneously, every other day. The primary outcome measures were
reduction in annual exacerbation rate and proportion of exacerbation-free
patients. At the end of the planned 2-year study, patients were offered re-
enrollment for an additional year to assess progression of disease, as
assessed by change in EDSS.

The results of this study, after 2 years, were that patients who received
8 MIU of interferon β had a significant reduction, by almost one-third, in the
annual exacerbation rate, as compared to placebo treated patients (0.84
vs. 1.27; $P = 0.0001$). More importantly, the degree of reduction in exacerbation rate was most impressive, almost 50%, in those exacerbations rated
as moderate or severe. The other primary end-point, proportion of patients
remaining exacerbation free, also showed a significant difference, favoring
interferon β (8 MIU interferon β = 36, placebo = 18, $P = 0.007$). The median
time to first exacerbation was significantly prolonged, nearly twice as long
in the 8 MIU group as compared to placebo ($P = 0.015$). Further, there
were significant reductions in the number and days of hospitalization and
need for steroids in the interferon β treated group. The interferon beta
1.6 MIU group demonstrated a dose–response effect, with clinical values
between that of the 8 MIU group and the placebo group in most outcome
measures.

The patients in this study had baseline and yearly MRI scans which were
analyzed in blinded fashion at one study site. MRI activity was assessed by
measuring new or enlarging lesions in a subset of 52 patients who had
scans every 6 weeks for 2 years. MRI activity was reduced in the interferon
β 8 MIU treatment group by 80% compared to the placebo group
($P = 0.0062$). The rate of new lesions, active lesions and number of patients
free of new lesions all significantly favored the interferon β 8 MIU group.
MRI lesion burden, measured on T2 weighted images, was significantly
less at 2 years in the treatment group ($P < 0.001$).

By the time all enrolled patients completed 3 years on protocol, the total
data set for the blinded, placebo controlled study included patients with a
median time on study of almost 4 years, including a few patients who completed 5 years. The analysis of the 3 year data and that for the entire data
set (all patients, all time on study) shows a continued significant decrease
in the relapse rate of about 30% ($P = 0.006$, pooled data, all patients, all
time points on study).[4] The same holds true for each individual year,

although significance was achieved individually only for the first 2 years, likely due to loss of power from successive dropouts in the later years. Progression of disease, assessed by the proportion of patients with a sustained worsening by 1 point on the EDSS, showed a trend, but not a significant difference, in favor of interferon β. The study was not powered to show a change in EDSS, but rather to assess change in relapse rate. The MRI data for all patients over the course of the study continued to show a dramatic effect from treatment with interferon β, with no significant increase in lesion burden through year five. The placebo group increased their T2 burden by about 10% per year. These data demonstrate a persistence of effect in the group response to interferon β (Figure 7.3).

The most common side effect of interferon β-1b was a flu-like syndrome characterized by fevers, chills, headache, and myalgias. This occurs shortly after injection and persists for a variable period, usually less than 24 hours. The flu-like syndrome wanes over weeks to months, but persists in up to 10% of patients. Rarely there are increases in liver enzymes (AST, ALT), which respond to dose reduction or drug discontinuation. Rare cases of liver disease have been attributed to interferon β. Redness at the injection sites is quite common and skin necrosis at the subcutaneous injection site is a rare occurrence.

Subsequently, interferon β-1b was tested in MS patients with secondary progressive disease. In a multicenter a double blind, randomized clinical trial conducted in Europe and published in 1998,[5] 718 secondary progressive MS (SPMS) patients with EDSS of 3–6.5 and at least two exacerbations

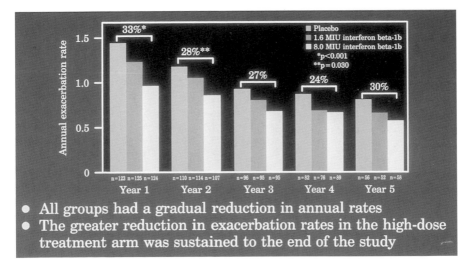

Figure 7.3
Interferon beta-1b: effect on annualized exacerbation rates.

in the prior 2 years were treated with either interferon β-1b, 8 MIU or placebo, planned for 3 years. The primary outcome measure was time to a sustained worsening of 1 point on the EDSS score (0.5 points if baseline EDSS was greater than 5.5). The study was stopped shortly prior to the planned ending because of overwhelming evidence of efficacy. The results reveal that the interferon treated group had a 22% reduction in rate of progression, which translated to a 12-month delay until reaching similar disability levels (Figure 7.4). Similarly, time to becoming wheelchair bound, EDSS ≥ 7, was delayed by 9 months. There was a significant reduction in the relapse rate in interferon treated patients and reduced MRI activity as measured by gadolinium enhancing lesions. There was also a significant reduction in both T2 and T1 lesion load and a lesser degree of NAA signal loss (a measure of neuronal/axonal loss) on MR spectroscopy. However, there was not a significant reduction in the development of cerebral atrophy, the cause for which has been speculated upon.

A second study of interferon β-1b in SPMS was conducted in North America with 939 patients with evidence of progression over the prior 2 years, but no relapse requirement. In this double blind, controlled trial patients received either placebo, interferon β-1b, 8 MIU, or interferon β-1b, 5 MIU/m^2 (which averaged 9.6 MIU for the entire group) subcutaneously every other day. The primary outcome measure was the same as in the European Interferon β-1b SP study. This planned 3-year study was stopped early for inability to achieve a significant difference in the primary outcome measure. As opposed to the European interferon β-1b SP study,

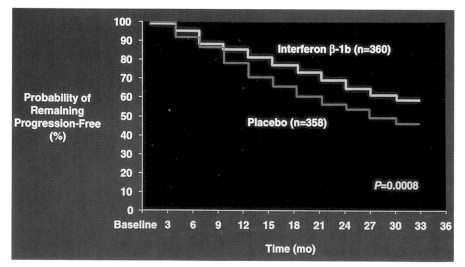

Figure 7.4
Interferon beta-1b (Betaferon): European Phase III trial in SPMS showed significant effect of the drug on slowing progression.

this study did not show a significant difference in disability measures between the treated groups and the placebo group. There were significant differences in reduction in relapse rate and MRI measures of activity and burden of disease (T2 lesion load).

There has been considerable speculation as to why the North American and European SP trials produced such different results. At entry, the EDSS scores were similar (5.1). There were several differences in the baseline demographics of the two populations. The North American study patients were older, had MS for a longer time and, perhaps most importantly, had fewer relapses and fewer gadolinium enhancing lesions, prior to study entry. The latter difference could indicate that the European SP population had a greater inflammatory element to their disease, and thus might respond better to an anti-inflammatory agent such as interferon β-1b. However, in the European study the interferon β-1b treated group had a significant reduction in MRI T1 black hole lesion load and improved MR spectroscopic analysis of NAA, both indicating less axonal damage. A better understanding of the causes for the disparity in these study results may materialize as our knowledge of the underlying pathogenic mechanisms of progressive disease increases.

Interferon β-1a

The pivotal trial of interferon β-1a (Avonex) in the United States comprised 301 patients with relapsing MS, who had at least two exacerbations over the prior 3 years and had an EDSS score between 1 and 3.5. Patients were assigned randomly to receive interferon, 6 MIU (30 μg) or a placebo via intramuscular (IM) injection, once weekly.[6] The trial was designed to last 2 years but was terminated prematurely because there were fewer dropouts than anticipated and as a result only 57% of the enrolled patients completed 2 years, and 77% completed 18 months. The primary outcome measure was the time to sustained progression of disability of at least 1 point on the EDSS, confirmed at 6 months (to lessen the chance that changes in EDSS were the result of exacerbations). A number of clinical and MRI measures served as secondary outcomes. The primary outcome measure was achieved with a 37% reduction in disability progression; 22% of patients receiving interferon progressed by 1 or more points while 35% of placebo patients progressed ($P = 0.02$) (Figure 7.5). In addition, there was a significant reduction in the annualized relapse rate for all patients, all time on study and especially for those treated for the full 2 years (18% all patients, all time on study and 32% for those completing 2 years). In relation to MRI there was a significant treatment effect on annual gadolinium enhanced MRI, a measure of disease activity, but the effect on total lesion volume did not reach statistical significance at 2 years. The side effect profile of interferon included flu-like symptoms (61% interferon vs. 40% placebo), muscle aches (34% vs. 15%), fever (23% vs. 13%), chills (21%

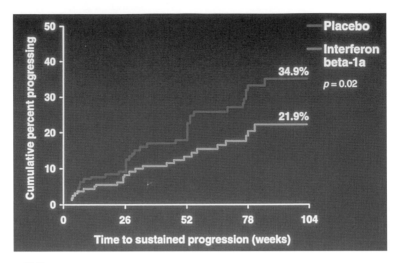

Figure 7.5
Interferon beta-1a: time to increased disability by ≥ 1 EDSS steps.

vs. 7%), with no differences found for headache, pain, or weaknesses. Overall, the agent was very well tolerated. This drug has now been approved by the FDA and is widely used in the United States. Subsequent analyses reveal a reduction in rate of development of cerebral atrophy and beneficial effects on cognition.

Preliminary results of a study of interferon β-1a (IMPACT Trial) in SPMS have been released. The study utilized a double dose, 60 μg, of interferon, given once weekly for 2 years to 436 patients with SPMS in the United States and Canada. The entry criteria were SPMS that had progressed over the past year in patients with an EDSS of 3.5–6.5 and an MRI consistent with MS. The primary outcome measure was a change in the Multiple Sclerosis Functional Composite (MSFC), a new outcome measure that was designed to be more sensitive to change than the EDSS. The initial report is of a slowing of progression, as measured by the MSFC, by 27% in patients treated with interferon β-1a compared to placebo patients. Analysis of other outcome measures is awaited. Equally as important will be the comparison of older outcome measures, such as the EDSS, with the MSFC, as this is the first study to utilize this scale as a primary outcome measure.

Another study with the Avonex form of interferon β-1a sought to determine whether treating individuals who suffered a single attack of demyelination (clinically isolated syndrome) would be less likely to develop a second, and therefore MS defining, attack if treated with interferon at a dose of 30 μg, IM, once weekly (CHAMPS Study).[7] This randomized, double blind study enrolled 383 patients who suffered a single event of either optic neuritis, brainstem/cerebellar dysfunction, or acute myelitis, and had two or more abnormalities consistent with demyelination on their MRI scan of the brain. Patients had to be screened within 2 weeks of symptom onset and were initially treated with IV methylprednisolone, 1 g daily for 3 days, followed by an oral prednisone taper. The study ran for nearly 3 years and demonstrated a reduced risk of having a second attack of 44% in those treated with interferon β-1a (approximately 50% of placebo treated patients had a second attack compared to approximately 35% of those treated with interferon β-1a) (Figure 7.6). There was a favorable effect of treatment on MRI metrics as well.

Another clinical trial of interferon β-1a (Rebif, Prisms Trial), from a different company (Ares Serono) consisted of a multicenter placebo controlled study of 560 patients with RRMS and Kurtzke scores of 0–5.0, who were randomized into a placebo group, 6 MIU (22 µg) or 12 MIU (44 µg) interferon β-1a, administered subcutaneously three times weekly for 2 years.[8] The results of this study were that patients in both treatment groups performed significantly better than placebo treated patients in respect to reduction in relapse rate (the primary outcome measure; 27% and 33% reductions for the 22 µg and 44 µg groups respectively), percentage of

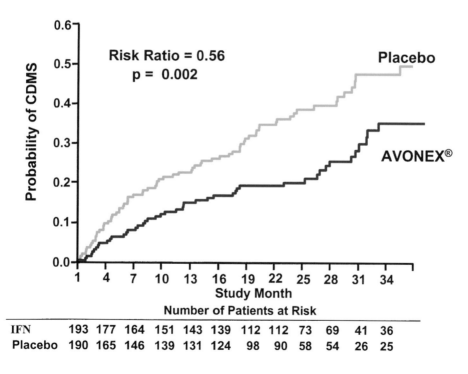

					Number of Patients at Risk						
IFN	193	177	164	151	143	139	112	112	73	69	41	36
Placebo	190	165	146	139	131	124	98	90	58	54	26	25

Figure 7.6

The CHAMPS trial of patients with clinically isolated syndromes showed a 44% reduction in conversion to clinically definite MS in patients taking interferon beta-1a (as Avonex®) compared to those taking placebo.

patients relapse free, time to first relapse, number of moderate or severe attacks, steroid use, and hospitalizations. Time to confirmed progression of disability by an increase in 1 point on the Kurtzke scale was also better in the treated groups. Analysis of MRI scans in the groups revealed decreased activity and lesion burden in the interferon treated patients. Although the higher dose group did better, there were no significant differences in the major clinical outcome measures between the two dosing groups (Figure 7.7).

A trial of this form of interferon β-1a (Rebif) in SPMS (SPECTRIMS Trial) has been completed.[9] This trial enrolled 618 patients in Europe and Canada, with SPMS, an EDSS of 3–6.5, a history of progressive deterioration for at least 6 months with an increase in EDSS of 1 or more points over the prior 2 years (0.5 points if the EDSS was 6 or 6.5), and a score of 2 or more in the pyramidal functional score. Patients were treated with interferon β-1a at either 22 or 44 μg, or placebo, subcutaneously, three times weekly for 3 years. The primary endpoint was time to onset of confirmed progression of 1 point on the EDSS. The results were that the study did not show a significant difference between the treated groups and placebo in the primary outcome measure, with results similar to those of the North American Interferon β-1b study. On further analysis of the patient

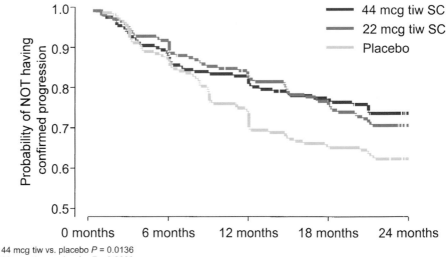

44 mcg tiw vs. placebo P = 0.0136
22 mcg tiw vs. placebo P = 0.0398
PRISMS Study Group. *Lancet* 1998; 352:1498–1504.

Figure 7.7
The PRISMS trial showed that patients receiving interferon beta-1a (as Rebif®) three times a week were statistically significantly less likely to progress than patents receiving placebo during the two years of the trial.

population, there was a suggestion of a better result in patients who had more relapses, again suggesting that relapsing forms of SPMS respond better than the nonrelapsing group. There were significant treatment effects seen for interferon β-1a in secondary outcomes such as relapse rate and MRI lesion load.

Another trial with the Rebif form of interferon β-1a studied the effect of treating patients with clinically probable or laboratory supported definite MS; i.e. early demyelinating disease (ETOMS Study).[10] Patients were seen within 3 months of symptom onset and had to have an MRI consistent with demyelinating disease. 308 patients were randomized to treatment with either placebo or the Rebif form of interferon β-1a, 22 μg subcutaneously once weekly. The entry criteria for this study complemented, rather then paralleled, those of the CHAMPS study in that this patient group included both monosymptomatic and polysymptomatic patients, with a longer latency from onset of symptoms to entry into the study. The dose of interferon utilized was lower than that used in CHAMPS. The result of the ETOMS study was that those treated with interferon were 24% less likely to develop a second attack. MRI metrics were also favorably affected by use of interferon.

Both ETOMS and CHAMPS provide data as to the effects of early treatment of demyelinating disease, prior to a definitive diagnosis of MS. However, the effect is modest; 35% of those treated with interferon in CHAMPS had a second attack within 3 years and, perhaps more importantly, 50% of the placebo treated patients did not have a second attack during the same period. Further, the longer term benefits of treatment were not assessed in these studies, nor the effect on disability. Longer term data will be needed to better define those patients who would benefit from complex therapy after a single attack and to separate these patients from those with monosymptomatic illnesses such as acute disseminated encephalomyelitis.

Interferon Dosing Issues

There has not been a prospective, well-designed study to determine the optimal dose of IFN. There has been considerable speculation about floor and ceiling dosing issues, but little data, especially as to maximal dosage. In the original IFN beta-1b study, a low dose (50 mcg) did not fare as well as the higher (250 mcg) dose. In the PRISMS trial, there were trends for better outcome with the higher dose that became more apparent during the subsequent open label extension. There has been a large, well-controlled study of IFN beta-1a given at single dose (30 mcg) and double dose (60 mcg), IM once weekly, which did not demonstrate any significant dosing effect. More recently, two studies, both open-label, have compared dosing across product lines. The EVIDENCE trial compared IFN beta-1a, 30 mcg IM once weekly, to 44 mcg SC three times weekly in relapsing MS patients. The examiners were blinded as to treatment. The primary outcome measure was percentage relapse free at 24 weeks. There were significantly more relapse free patients in the higher dose IFN beta-1a (three times weekly) group than in the once weekly group (74.9% v. 63.3; p<0.001). There was also a significant reduction in the number of new MRI abnormalities seen. At 48 weeks, the higher dosed group continued to have significantly fewer exacerbations, but there was little difference seen between the two groups in the second 24 week period (unpublished data, obtained from the FDA web page-http://www.fda.gov/cber/review/ifnbser030702r1.pdf). A second comparative study is the INCOMIN trial, which compared IFN beta-1a, 30 mcg IM weekly to IFN beta-1b, 250 mcg SC every other day. The study was open-label and randomized. The primary outcome measures were number of relapse free patients and number of patients without new T2 lesions at two years. The unpublished results, as presented by the lead investigator, demonstrated a significant benefit favoring the higher dose and frequency of IFN for both primary outcome measures (percentage relapse free- IFN beta-1a 36%, IFN beta-1b 51%; new T2 lesion free- IFN beta-1a 26%, IFN beta-1b 55%) as well as several secondary outcome measures. Additional data on dosing, especially directed toward higher doses, prospective, long term and fully blinded will be of value in resolving these dosing and frequency of administration issues.

Glatiramer acetate

There were two trials of glatiramer acetate (GA, Copaxone) in RRMS in the United States. The first comprised 48 patients with at least two exacerbations in the prior 2 years and an EDSS score less than 6. Patients received GA 20 mg or placebo subcutaneously, daily for 2 years.[11] This study showed a reduction of 75% in relapse rate (0.6 relapses per year in the GA group compared to 2.4 relapses with placebo). There also was a slowing of the rate of progression of disability.

The second trial utilized 251 RRMS patients with at least two exacerbations in the prior 2 years and an EDSS score of 0–5. They received either GA 20 mg or placebo subcutaneously (SC) daily for 2 years.[12] The primary outcome measure was a difference in relapse rate. This study was planned to last 2 years but was extended, maintaining the double blind, placebo controlled design through 35 months.[13] The primary outcome measure, reduction in relapse rate, was better in the GA treated group at 2 years and also at 35 months (at 2 years the rates were: 1.19% (annualized rate 0.6) for GA compared to 1.68 (annualized rate 0.84) for placebo, a 29% reduction, $P = 0.007$). Other outcome measures, e.g. percentage of patients improved or worsened, also favored GA. There were no organized MRI data obtained in this trial. Open label extension data demonstrated long term efficacy and the rather disconcerting finding that patients who were initially randomized to placebo group never caught up to the patients treated with GA from onset, as assessed by EDSS (Figure 7.8).

A subsequent 9-month MRI based study in Europe and Canada of 239 RRMS patients with at least one gadolinium enhancing lesion demonstrated that GA, 20 mg SC, daily, decreased MRI activity and lesion load over time, but does so more slowly and less extensively than seen with interferon, suggesting a different mechanism of action for these two agents.[14] The GA effect on enhancing lesions was not apparent until after 4 months, while the effect from interferon occurs within weeks of initiation. The effect on lesion load in the GA study followed a similar time course as the enhancing lesions, which is not that different from that seen with interferon. Of interest, by the end of the study, at 9 months, there was a significant reduction in relapse rate in the GA treated patients of 33%.

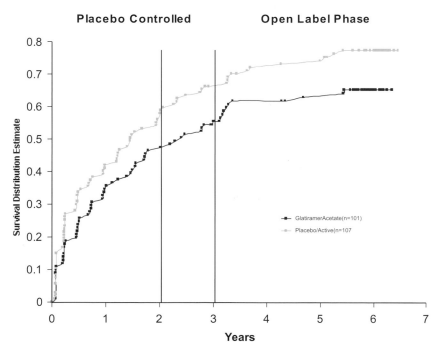

Placebo Controlled   **Open Label Phase**

Legend:
■ GlatiramerAcetate(n=101)
□ Placebo/Active(n=107)

Y-axis: Survival Distribution Estimate
X-axis: Years

Figure 7.8
Effect of glatiramer acetate and placebo on disability, as measured by EDSS during the randomized, double-blind, placebo-controlled trial, the blinded extension phase, and the open-label continuation.

Antibodies

The role of neutralizing antibodies to the disease-modifying therapies has been difficult to determine and more difficult to integrate into clinical practice. In the North American RRMS interferon β-1b study, the initial analysis revealed that approximately 35% of patients developed neutralizing antibodies (NAB) over 2 years and the beneficial effect on relapses was diminished in those patients.[15] A subsequent reanalysis, using a different assay and different statistical approach, did not confirm this result. Long term follow-up suggests that most patients that develop NAB will lose them over time. NAB did not appear to be a problem in the interferon β-1b SPMS study. Neutralizing antibodies were reported in 22% of patients in the initial RRMS interferon β-1a (Avonex) study at 24 months. The effect of the antibodies on clinical and MRI end points did not appear to reach significance; however, the numbers involved were small as a result of the early termination of the study and there was some concern about the reliability of the assay. The results were re-evaluated using another antibody assay and revealed a considerably lower incidence of antibodies. In the other RR interferon β-1a (Rebif) study, the lower dose had a higher incidence of NAB and there appeared to be a lessened efficacy in antibody positive patients.[16] The results from these studies are not directly comparable, as different assays and different standards were employed. Further, there are data to suggest that interferon antibodies disappear over time.[17] There are good data to suggest that the NAB that develop cross-react with any of the interferon preparations and natural interferon as well. The same issues that hamper full interpretation of the data cloud the use of NAB determinations in clinical practice. Some patients will seem to do quite well on interferon despite NAB and some patients do not appear to benefit from interferon despite the absence of NAB. Treatment-altering decisions should rest primarily on the clinical picture, despite the absence of a well accepted definition of clinical failure. The presence of NAB, at high titer, on more than one occasion, in a patient who is not doing well, could suggest that a noninterferon treatment alternative should be pursued. There is no evidence for neutralizing antibodies in GA patients.

Mitoxantrone

The first agent to be approved in the United States for use in SPMS was mitoxantrone (Novantrone), approved in 2000 for treatment of what is now referred to as worsening forms of relapsing MS, i.e., patients with RRMS, SPMS or progressive-relapsing MS (PRMS) who were rapidly deteriorating. This agent was not tested in primary progressive MS (PPMS) patients. Mitoxantrone is a cytotoxic anthracenedione with potent immunosuppressive actions. The pivotal study of mitoxantrone was performed in Europe as a multicenter, observer blinded, placebo controlled trial of 194 patients randomized to receive either placebo, mitoxantrone 5 mg/m^2 or mito-xantrone 12 mg/m^2 IV every 3 months for 2 years. Patients had to have an EDSS of 3–6 and to have deteriorated by at least 1 point in the prior 18 months. The primary outcome measure was a multivariate analysis of five measures – change in mean EDSS from baseline to month 24, change in ambulation index, number of corticosteroid-treated exacerbations, time to first relapse, and change in the Standard Neurological Status (a propri-etary scale utilized at some centers in Europe) in the 12 mg/m^2 group com-pared to placebo. Once the multivariate analysis was shown to be positive, the individual components were to be analysed. This type of analysis has not been used in other MS studies. The results for the 12 mg/m^2 group, the intended dosing arm, were significantly better compared to placebo. Similar results were seen in the individual components of this analysis. The 5 mg/m^2 dose gave intermediate results, except for the change in mean EDSS, where it was better than the larger dose. In the secondary outcome measures, the percentage of patients with a confirmed change in EDSS by 1 point was 64% better in the 12 mg/m^2 group as compared to placebo. There was a 69% reduction in annualized relapse rate, but these data, although impressive by current standards, must be viewed with some circumspection, as an unblinded physician made the determination of relapse. MRI measures were of activity (gadolinium enhancing lesions) and lesion load on T2 weighted scans. The study continued to evaluate patients after the 2-year dosing period and at the end of 3 years, there was still evidence of a treatment effect. These results have not yet been published.

Another multicenter European study compared the combination of mitoxantrone 20 mg IV and IV methylprednisolone to IV methylpred-nisolone alone, given monthly for 6 months.[18] The 42 patients entered were RRMS or SPMS with an EDSS of 6 or less and active disease on one of two baseline scans. The primary endpoint was the proportion of patients with-out new enhancing lesions. There was an 86% reduction in the proportion of patients with new disease activity on the mitoxantrone/methylpred-nisolone group as compared to the methylprednisolone alone group by month six. Secondary endpoints included a reduction in relapse rate in the combined group.

The major toxicity of mitoxantrone is cardiac. There is a cumulative dose related cardiotoxicity which limits lifetime exposure. Current recommenda-tions are for use up to a cumulative dosage of 140 mg/m^2. The potential for adverse cardiac events is increased in those with prior exposure to other cardiotoxic cytotoxic agents or mediastinal radiation. The cardiac toxicity data comes from patients with tumors and the potential for cardiac prob-lems in an MS population is, as yet, unknown, and not encountered in the above trials. Pretreatment cardiac output screening is advised and moni-toring should occur after each dose beyond a cumulative exposure of 100 mg/m^2. Other side effects include allopecia, menstrual irregularity, amenorrhea, and leukopenia. None of these was particularly severe. The issue of secondary leukemia is still open, although remote.

Mitoxantrone has been approved for use in worsening RRMS, SPMS, and PR MS patients. In general, this agent should be saved for patients with aggressive disease, especially if they have failed interferon or GA, keeping in mind that there is a limit to the total dose that can be administered. The data from the above studies is the most impressive of any chemotherapeutic agent (see below).

Other agents for which there are less compelling data for efficacy

Cyclophosphamide

There have been a number of studies of cyclophosphamide treatment of progressive MS.[19,20] Some studies have suggested a benefit, while others have not. Comparison between trials is always hazardous, and various induction protocols have been utilized, some with the addition of steroids and/or plasmapheresis. The Canadian Cooperative Study provides the most convincing evidence for a lack of efficacy. Nevertheless, there are many anecdotes of success leading to use of this agent in desperate cases.

Azathioprine

Azathioprine has been studied in several clinical trials.[21–23] A modest effect on relapses has been shown, but no convincing effect on progressive disease. Despite this, azathioprine is probably the commonest cytostatic agent utilized in progressive MS, again primarily in desperation and anecdotally. Systemic toxicity is an important consideration with this agent, although less than with cyclophosphamide.

Methotrexate

Methotrexate has been utilized in other autoimmune diseases, e.g. rheumatoid arthritis (RA). A study of patients with progressive MS was carried out using a dosing regimen similar to that used in RA, 7.5 mg orally per week.[24] This double blind, placebo controlled study revealed a modest beneficial effect of methotrexate on a composite scale. Benefit was found on a measure of upper extremity function, but no effect was seen on ambulation. Toxicity was minimal.

Cladribine

This antineoplastic agent is approved for treatment of hairy cell leukemia. Pilot studies suggested a benefit in RRMS and progressive MS patients. A larger, multicenter trial in a patients with both primary progressive and secondary progressive MS did not demonstrate any clinical benefit after 1 year, but did show a marked reduction in gadolinium enhancing MRI lesions.[25] Effects on other MRI measures were unimpressive. Toxicity was acceptable.

Cyclosporine

Cyclosporine, an immunosuppressant agent commonly used in transplant recipients, was studied in progressive MS. The therapeutic effect was quite modest and there was significant toxicity, primarily hypertension and renal toxicity.[26]

Repetitive courses of steroids

There is no demonstrated role for chronic administration of corticosteroids in MS and considerable potential morbidity. Some have advocated the periodic use of pulses of steroids in secondary progressive disease, rather than just using pulses for acute exacerbations. The only tested approach involved treatment of progressive MS patients with high dose methylprednisolone, IV every other month for up to 2 years. There was no convincing effect of this treatment approach.[27]

Total lymphoid irradiation (TLI)

TLI has been used to induce immunosuppression, primarily through lymphopenia. When used alone or in combination with low dose corticosteroids, the course of progressive MS can be slowed temporarily. The results are best when accompanied by lymphopenia. This is a complex therapy, which is still investigational and best performed at selected centers with specific expertise.

IVIg

IVIg has been tested in RRMS in a double blind placebo controlled trial of 148 patients in Austria.[28] Patients had to have had at least two documented exacerbations in the prior 2 years and an EDSS of 1–6. Patients were randomized to receive either placebo or IVIg 0.15–0.2 g/kg body weight monthly for 2 years. The primary outcome measure was change in EDSS. IVIg treatment had a significant, albeit modest, effect on mean EDSS and a categorical measure of change. There was also a 59% reduction in relapse rate. The agent was well tolerated. There were no MRI data collected.

A study of 26 patients with either RRMS ($n = 21$) or SPMS ($n = 5$) was conducted in Denmark,[29] with difference in gadolinium enhancing lesions as the primary outcome measure. Utilizing a crossover design, patients were treated with IVIg 2 g/kg (1 g/kg daily for 2 days) or placebo monthly for 6 months. There was a significant reduction in new and total gadolinium enhancing lesions in patients while on IVIg. Although the reduction in relapse rate was not significant, the number of patients relapse free was. There were more side effects than seen in other IVIg studies, likely related to the higher dosing schedule.

Another study of IVIg was conducted in Israel with 40 patients with RRMS.[30] Patients were randomized to receive either placebo or IVIg 0.4 g/kg/day for 5 days then 0.4 g/kg every 2 months for 2 years. There was a significant reduction in relapse rate and increased number of exacerbation free patients, the primary outcome measures, in IVIg patients. MRI measures were not significantly different. Treatment was well tolerated.

The data on use of IVIg in MS are not yet compelling, but certainly intriguing. Unfortunately, the optimal dose is not clear from the current studies. A large, well designed European study of IVIg, 1 g/kg monthly, in SPMS, has recently concluded and failed to show any effect on disease activity. Other studies are planned.

Bone marrow/stem cell transplantation

There are several anecdotal reports of the use of these techniques in MS, but no controlled data. Absent controlled trials, single case studies and even multiple cases, with an international registry, are unlikely to yield convincing data. There is a definable morbidity, and, thus far, rather worrisome mortality associated with this procedure in MS patients.

References

1. Rose AS, Kuzma JW, Kurtzke JF, Namerow NS, Sibley WA, Tourtellotte WW. Cooperative study in the evaluation of therapy in multiple sclerosis. ACTH. Neurology 1970; 20:1–59.

2. Miller DM, Weinstock-Guttman B, Bethoux F, et al. A meta-analysis of methylprednisolone in recovery from multiple sclerosis exacerbations. Mult Scler 2000; 6:267–273.

3. IFNB Multiple Sclerosis Study Group. Interferon β-1b is effective in relapsing-remitting multiple sclerosis. I. Clinical results of a multicenter, randomized, double-blind, placebo-controlled trial. Neurology 1993; 43:655–661.

4. The IFNB Multiple Sclerosis Study Group and The University of British Columbia MS/MRI Analysis Group. Interferon β-1b in the treatment of multiple sclerosis: final outcome of the randomized controlled trial. Neurology 1995; 45:1277–1285.

5. European Study Group on Interferon β-1b in Secondary Progressive MS. Placebo-con-trolled multicentre randomised trial of interferon β-1b in treatment of secondary progressive multiple sclerosis. Lancet 1998; 352: 1491–1497.

6. Jacobs LD, Cookfair DL, Rudick RA, et al. Intramuscular interferon β-1a for disease progression in relapsing multiple sclerosis. The Multiple Sclerosis Collaborative Research Group (MSCRG). Ann Neurol 1996; 39:285–294.

7. Jacobs LD, Beck RW, Simon JH, et al. Intramuscular interferon β-1a therapy initiated during a first demyelinating event in multiple sclerosis. CHAMPS Study Group. N Engl J Med 2000; 343:898–904.

8. PRISMS (Prevention of Relapses and Disability by Interferon β-1a Subcutaneously in Multiple Sclerosis) Study Group. Randomised double-blind placebo-controlled study of interferon β-1a in relapsing/remitting multiple sclerosis. Lancet 1998; 352:1498–1504.

9. Secondary Progressive Efficacy Clinical Trial of Recombinant

Interferon-β-1a in MS (SPECTRIMS) Study Group. Randomized controlled trial of interferon β-1a in secondary progressive MS: clinical results. Neurology 2001; 56:1496–1504.

10. Comi G, Filippi M, Barkhof F, et al. Effect of early interferon treatment on conversion to definite multiple sclerosis: a randomised study. Lancet 2001; 357:1576–1582.

11. Bornstein MB, Miller A, Slagle S, et al. A pilot trial of Cop 1 in exacerbating-remitting multiple sclerosis. N Engl J Med 1987; 317:408–414.

12. Johnson KP, Brooks BR, Cohen JA, et al. Copolymer 1 reduces relapse rate and improves disability in relapsing-remitting multiple sclerosis: results of a phase III multicenter, double-blind placebo-controlled trial. The Copolymer 1 Multiple Sclerosis Study Group. Neurology 1995; 45:1268–1276.

13. Johnson KP, Brooks BR, Cohen JA, et al. Extended use of glatiramer acetate (Copaxone) is well tolerated and maintains its clinical effect on multiple sclerosis relapse rate and degree of disability. Copolymer 1 Multiple Sclerosis Study Group. Neurology 1998; 50:701–708.

14. Comi G, Filippi M, Wolinsky JS. European/Canadian multicenter, double-blind, randomized, placebo-controlled study of the effects of glatiramer acetate on magnetic resonance imaging – measured disease activity and burden in patients with relapsing multiple sclerosis. European/Canadian Glatiramer Acetate Study Group. Ann Neurol 2001; 49:290–297.

15. The IFNB Multiple Sclerosis Study Group and The University of British Columbia MS/MRI Analysis Group. Neutralizing antibodies during treatment of multiple sclerosis with interferon β-1b: experience during the first three years. Neurology 1996; 47:889–894.

16. The PRISMS (Prevention of Relapses and Disability by Interferon-β-1a Subcutaneously in Multiple Sclerosis) Study Group and the University of British Columbia MS/MRI Analysis Group. PRISMS-4: long-term efficacy of interferon-β-1a in relapsing MS. Neurology 2001; 56:1628–1636.

17. Rice GP, Paszner B, Oger J, Lesaux J, Paty D, Ebers G. The evolution of neutralizing antibodies in multiple sclerosis patients treated with interferon β-1b. Neurology 1999; 52:1277–1279.

18. Edan G, Miller D, Clanet M, et al. Therapeutic effect of mitoxantrone combined with methylprednisolone in multiple sclerosis: a randomised multicentre study of active disease using MRI and clinical criteria. J Neurol Neurosurg Psychiatry 1997; 62:112–118.

19. The Canadian Cooperative Multiple Sclerosis Study Group. The Canadian Cooperative Trial of Cyclophosphamide and Plasma Exchange in Progressive Multiple Sclerosis. Lancet 1991; 337:441–446.

20. Hauser SL, Dawson DM, Lehrich JR, et al. Intensive immunosuppression in progressive multiple sclerosis. A randomized, three-arm study of high-dose intravenous cyclophosphamide, plasma exchange, and ACTH. N Engl J Med 1983; 308:173–180.

21. Goodkin DE, Bailly RC, Teetzen ML, Hertsgaard D, Beatty WW. The efficacy of azathioprine in relapsing-remitting multiple sclerosis. Neurology 1991; 41:20–25.

22. Ellison GW, Myers LW, Mickey MR, et al. A placebo-controlled, randomized, double-masked, variable dosage, clinical trial of azathioprine with and without methylprednisolone in multiple

sclerosis. Neurology 1989; 39:1018–1026.

23. Anonymous. Double-masked trial of azathioprine in multiple sclerosis. British and Dutch Multiple Sclerosis Azathioprine Trial Group. Lancet 1988; ii:179–183.

24. Goodkin DE, Rudick RA, VanderBrug MS, Daughtry MM, Van D. Low-dose oral methotrexate in chronic progressive multiple sclerosis: analyses of serial MRIs. Neurology 1996; 47:1153–1157.

25. Rice GP, Filippi M, Comi G. Cladribine and progressive MS: clinical and MRI outcomes of a multicenter controlled trial. Cladribine MRI Study Group. Neurology 2000; 54:1145–1155.

26. The Multiple Sclerosis Study Group. Efficacy and toxicity of cyclosporine in chronic progressive multiple sclerosis: a randomized, double-blinded, placebo-controlled clinical trial. Ann Neurol 1990; 27:591–605.

27. Goodkin DE, Kinkel RP, Weinstock-Guttman B, et al. A phase II study of i.v. methylprednisolone in secondary-progressive multiple sclerosis. Neurology 1998; 51:239–245.

28. Fazekas F, Deisenhammer F, Strasser-Fuchs S, Nahler G, Mamoli B. Randomised placebo-controlled trial of monthly intravenous immunoglobulin therapy in relapsing-remitting multiple sclerosis. Austrian Immunoglobulin in Multiple Sclerosis Study Group. Lancet 1997; 349(9052):589–593.

29. Sorensen PS, Wanscher B, Jensen CV, et al. Intravenous immunoglobulin G reduces MRI activity in relapsing multiple sclerosis. Neurology 1998; 50:1273–1281.

30. Achiron A, Barak Y, Goren M, et al. Intravenous immune globulin in multiple sclerosis: clinical and neuroradiological results and implications for possible mechanisms of action. Clin Exp Immunol 1996; 104(suppl 1):67–70.

8
Symptomatic treatments

Overview

MS patients experience symptoms which limit daily activities, interfere with personal and professional relationships, and lower self esteem (Table 8.1). These symptoms often have significant impact on quality of life. Their management is a major goal of MS therapy, regardless of a patient's age, gender, disease duration, clinical subtype, or disease severity. In a recent survey symptoms were found to be undertreated in most patients.[1] Optimal symptom management provides a real opportunity to better the life of MS patients.[2]

Symptomatic treatment strategies can be divided into several major categories (Figure 8.1). When assessing patients it is helpful to have them rank their most bothersome symptoms, design a therapeutic plan for each one, and then address them in turn. This not only responds to the patient's priorities and needs, but also creates an organized plan for optimal symptom management. Management should be reassessed at regular intervals, since symptoms are dynamic and often fluctuate over time. They should be considered jointly, and not just in isolation, since comorbid symptoms influence each other.

Table 8.1 Frequent symptoms in MS.

- Fatigue
- Cognitive loss
- Depression
- Spasticity
- Pain and sensory disturbances
- Paroxysmal attacks
- Tremor
- Bladder disturbances
- Bowel dysfunction
- Sexual dysfunction
- Ambulation difficulties

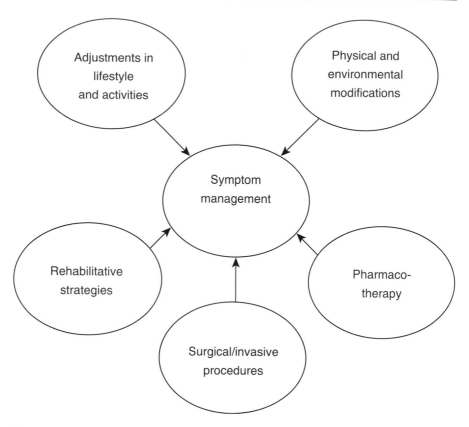

Figure 8.1
Symptomatic treatment strategies.

Fatigue

Fatigue may be the single most disabling symptom of MS.[3,4] It is experienced by up to 90% of patients, can be the presenting complaint of MS, can precede or be part of an acute relapse, or can occur in isolation. As an isolated symptom, however, it is not considered a relapse. MS patients experience several types of fatigue. There is normal fatigue, the fatigue of depression, fatigue due to disturbed sleep, fatigue as a side effect of medication, fatigue due to impaired mobility requiring greater effort, fatigue due to physical deconditioning, and primary fatigue. Primary MS fatigue is distinct from normal fatigue, and is a major reason for inability to work, even in patients with a relatively intact neurological examination. Primary fatigue does not require physical exertion, is not relieved by rest, and often comes on unprovoked in a wave that overcomes and debilitates the patient. It typically occurs daily, gets worse as the day progresses, comes on easily and is suddenly severe, and interferes with daily activities. A unique feature is that it is often aggravated by heat and humidity, and improved by cooling. Fatigue is subjective and therefore hard to define and measure. One proposed definition is the subjective lack of physical and/or mental energy that is perceived by the individual or caregiver to interfere with usual or desired activities.[5] Another definition is an overwhelming sense of tiredness, lack of energy, and feeling of exhaustion that is distinct from weakness or depression. MS fatigue can be acute, or chronic and persistent. When fatigue is present on at least half of the days, over a period of 6 weeks or longer, it is considered to be chronic.

The cause of MS fatigue is not understood.[6,7] Various theories suggest it represents impaired cortical circuitry, conduction block, increased energy demands for muscle activation, or a side effect of immune/inflammatory factors such as proinflammatory cytokines. Some studies report an association with subtle physiologic disturbances such as decreased firing of motor units, abnormal exercise related muscle activation and metabolism, and impaired drive to the motor cortex.[8,9] Although MS fatigue is not explained by excessive muscle fatigue, neuromuscular junction blockade, decreased central drive to motor neurons, or central motor pathway dysfunction, there are reported CNS disturbances.[6,10] A recent ^{12}F-fluorodeoxyglucose positron emission tomography study found frontal cortex and basal ganglia hypometabolism in fatigued MS patients, with compensatory hypermetabolism in the cerebellar vermis and anterior cingulate region.[11] Event-related potential studies show slowed reaction times in fatigued patients, consistent with disrupted intracortical circuitry.[12] For most patients multiple factors are likely involved. MS fatigue shows a consistent correlation with heat sensitivity, active disease, and decreased activity levels. There is inconsistent correlation with progressive disease, corticospinal tract involvement, and presence of depression, and no correlation with age, gender, disease duration, the neurological examination, severity of depression, or MRI disease parameters (total lesion burden, contrast lesion activity). Fatigue is one of the symptoms of depression. However, primary MS fatigue is clearly distinct from the fatigue of depression. Although it often occurs unprovoked, MS fatigue can certainly be brought on by physical activities. Physical deconditioning in and of itself can also contribute to this symptom, emphasizing that MS patients experience multiple types of fatigue (normal fatigue, primary MS fatigue, secondary fatigue due to deconditioning, overexertion fatigue, depression fatigue, unrelated fatigue).

There are a number of brief self-report rating scales to measure fatigue. A recent clinical practice guideline endorsed use of the Modified Fatigue Impact Scale (MFIS), from the MS Quality of Life Inventory (Figure 8.2).[5] This is likely to emerge as the preferred rating scale. It can be used to provide a more objective measure of response to treatment.

Assessment of primary MS fatigue is multidimensional (Table 8.2). It needs to be tailored to the individual, and may change over time. For example, fatigue is often worse during summer months, and may require

Fatigue is a feeling of physical tiredness and lack of energy that many people experience from time to time. But people who have medical conditions like MS experience stronger feelings of fatigue more often and with greater impact than others.

Following is a list of statements that describe the effects of fatigue. Please read each statement carefully, then *circle the one number* that best indicates how often fatigue has affected you in this way during the *past 4 weeks*. (If you need help in marking your responses, *tell the interviewer the number of the best response.*) *Please answer every question.* If you are not sure which answer to select, choose the one answer that comes closest to describing you. Ask the interviewer to explain any words or phrases that you do not understand.

Name _____   Date_____/_____/_____

ID# _____   Test 1 2 3 4

Because of my fatigue during the past 4 weeks…	Almost never	Rarely	Sometimes	Often	Always
1. I have been less alert.	0	1	2	3	4
2. I have had difficulty paying attention for long periods of time.	0	1	2	3	4
3. I have been unable to think clearly.	0	1	2	3	4
4. I have been clumsy and uncoordinated.	0	1	2	3	4
5. I have been forgetful.	0	1	2	3	4
6. I have had to pace myself in my physical activities.	0	1	2	3	4
7. I have been less motivated to do anything that requires physical effort.	0	1	2	3	4
8. I have been less motivated to participate in social activities.	0	1	2	3	4
9. I have been limited in my ability to do things away from home.	0	1	2	3	4
10. I have trouble maintaining physical effort for long periods	0	1	2	3	4
11. I have had difficulty making decisions.	0	1	2	3	4
12. I have been less motivated to do anything that requires thinking.	0	1	2	3	4
13. My muscles have felt weak.	0	1	2	3	4
14. I have been physically uncomfortable.	0	1	2	3	4
15. I have had trouble finishing tasks that require thinking	0	1	2	3	4
16. I have had difficulty organizing my thoughts when doing things at home or at work.	0	1	2	3	4
17. I have been less able to complete tasks that require physical effort.	0	1	2	3	4
18. My thinking has been slowed down.	0	1	2	3	4
19. I have had trouble concentrating.	0	1	2	3	4
20. I have limited my physical activities.	0	1	2	3	4
21. I have needed to rest more often or for longer periods.	0	1	2	3	4

Instructions for Scoring the MFIS
Items on the MFIS can be aggregated into three subscales (physical, cognitive, and psychosocial), as well as into a total MFIS score. All items are scaled so that higher scores indicate a greater impact of fatigue on a person's activities.

Physical Subscale
This scale can range from 0 to 36. It is computed by added raw scores on the following items 4+6+7+10+13+14+17+20+21.

Cognitive Subscale
This scale can range from 0 to 40. It is computed by added raw scores on the following items 1+2+3+5+11+12+15+16+18+19.

Psychosocial Subscale
This scale can range from 0 to 8. It is computed by added raw scores on the following items 8+9.

Total MFIS Score
The total MFIS score can range from 0 to 84. It is computed by adding scores on the physical, cognitive, and psychosocial subscales.

Figure 8.2
Modified fatigue impact scale (MFIS).

Table 8.2 Assessment of MS fatigue.

- Determine the extent, severity, and impact of the fatigue problem
  - Focused history
  - Interviews with associates

- Make sure fatigue problem not directly related to MS (tertiary fatigue)
  - Consider medical conditions such as thyroid disease, anemia, infection, malignancy, or a systemic disorder
  - Review the person's sleep patterns for poor sleep hygiene or a frank sleep disorder
  - Review all MS and non-MS drugs

- Consider whether fatigue is a consequence of their MS impairment/disability (secondary MS fatigue)
  - There is restricted mobility/use of assistive devices, with excessive effort requirements/deconditionizing fatigue
  - There are limitations in respiratory function

- Assess for fatigue due to MS (primary MS fatigue)
  - All other causes are excluded
  - Fatigue is temperature sensitive

- Assess for symptom comorbidity
  - Depression
  - Pain

more intense treatment during this season. Fatigue might need to be treated during the demanding work week, but not treated during the weekend when there is more opportunity to rest.

Although MS patients who complain of fatigue do not generally require an extensive workup, it is important to consider potential contributing factors such as an unrelated medical condition, iatrogenic drug effect, poor sleep hygiene, and the fatigue of depression. It is also important to distinguish secondary MS fatigue, which results from increased energy expenditure due to MS-related ambulation or respiratory difficulties. Treatment of fatigue must be multimodality (Table 8.3). Although fatigue occurs independent of depression and pain, these symptoms are frequently comorbidities and need to be treated to assure an optimal therapeutic response. Commonly used medications to treat MS fatigue are outlined in Table 8.4. Although amantadine (Symmetrel) remains first line therapy, modafinil (Provigil) is increasingly used.[13] Patients start at 100 mg daily, and can be increased to 200 mg (and as high as 400 mg) if response is suboptimal.

Cognitive abnormalities

Cognitive abnormalities are another major MS symptom. They are rarely prominent early, although in unusual cases dementia or psychiatric illness can be the presenting feature of MS. Cognitive abnormalities are reported

Table 8.3 Treatment of primary MS fatigue.

- Education and identification of types of fatigue, when they occur, precipitating factors
  - Primary
  - Secondary
  - Tertiary

- Correct fatigue due to comorbid conditions, poor sleep hygiene, iatrogenic causes

- Lifestyle changes
  - Schedule rest periods and naps
  - Rearrange activities in finite segments, during low fatigue times
  - Modify types of activities

- Environmental modifications
  - Cooling devices (cold drinks, loose clothing, cold compresses/showers, air conditioning, cooling devices)
  - Bedside commode
  - Workplace/home adjustments and modifications (moderate pace, comfortable position, organize area, optimal temperature)

- Rehabilitation strategies
  - Regular aerobic/endurance exercise program (40 minutes 3 times weekly)
  - Energy conservation techniques/simplification of work tasks (avoid lifting/carrying heavy objects, delegate stressful/fatiguing work, maintain good posture)
  - Use of assistive devices
  - Consider vocational retraining

- Psychological interventions
  - Acceptance of limitations
  - Behavioral techniques

- Pharmacotherapy
  - Amantadine (Symmetrel)
  - Modafinil (Provigil)
  - Pemoline (Cylert)
  - Fluoxetine (Prozac)
  - Amphetamines (Ritalin, Adderol, etc.)
  - 4 Aminopyridine (4AP)
  - Caffeine
  - Aspirin

in 13–72% of patient series, but on the average are seen in 43–46% of patients.[14,15] Some studies find that secondary progressive MS patients are the most likely clinical subset to have serious cognitive problems.[16,17] Cognitive deficits are severe enough to be considered dementia in about 10% of affected patients. Problems include cognitive loss, cognitive fatigue (deficits occur with continued effort), and behavioral changes.[18] MS involves specific cognitive domains (Table 8.5). Abnormalities can be subtle and overlooked by both physicians and patients. Family members may interpret cognitive difficulties as deliberate misbehavior or acting out.

Table 8.4 Major medications used to treat MS fatigue.

Drug	Dose	Mechanism of action	Comments
Amantadine	100 mg bid	Glutamate antagonist, dopamine releaser receptor, reuptake inhibitor agonist	Nausea, lightheadedness, nervousness, insomnia (5 –10%), impaired concentration
		↓ NMDA receptor acetylcholine release	Irritability, depression, confusion, hallucinations, delusions, paranoia, seizures, livedo reticularis, headache, peripheral edema, constipation, dry mouth (1–5%)
		Antiviral agent	
			Psychosis, urinary retention, corneal opacities (< 1%)
Modafinil	100–400 mg (qd)	Activation of hypothalamus, medial forebrain	Headache, nausea, anxiety/nervousness, dry mouth, insomnia
Pemoline	18.75–112.5 mg (qd)	CNS stimulant (amphetamine-like)	Rare hepatotoxicity (monitor liver enzymes), aplastic anemia
			Insomnia (a.m. dosing), anorexia, irritability, weight loss, GI symptoms, palpitations
Fluoxetine	20–80 mg (qd)	Selective serotonin reuptake inhibitor, antidepressant	Anorexia, weight loss, anxiety
			Insomnia, drowsiness
			Tremor, GI symptoms

Table 8.5 Cognitive domains affected in MS.

- Attention
- Memory (short and long term)
- Information processing speed
- Abstract reasoning (problem solving, conceptual reasoning)
- Visuospatial perception
- Learning

The brief repeatable battery of neuropsychological tests, which is shorter than the typical neurocognitive evaluation, has been developed specifically for MS. It consists of five tests (selective reminding test, 10/36 spatial recall test, symbol digit modalities test, paced auditory serial addition test, word list generation test), and is available in two parallel versions (A and B).[19]

Cognitive difficulties produce significant disability.[17,20] Patients are less likely to be employed, and to engage in social and vocational activities. They have more sexual dysfunction, greater problems with activities of daily living, and greater psychopathology. Some patients show changes in mood and personality, with relatively preserved intellect and language function. Cognitive loss in MS does not correlate with physical disability, fatigue, or depression. There are correlations with neuroimaging parameters of cortical/subcortical involvement.[17,21–27] Increasing lesion burden, along with loss of brain volume (including neurons and axons), appears to ultimately disrupt sufficient interneuronal circuitry to result in cognitive loss. Cognitive deficits have been associated with abnormal event-related potentials such as P300, and hypometabolic disturbances on positron emission tomography.[28]

When cognitive problems are suspected in MS, patients should be formally evaluated. Both patients and families need to be educated about expected difficulties and coping mechanisms. Computer assisted cognitive retraining may be of benefit.[29] The best current treatment for cognitive loss is probably preventive, using strategies to minimize lesion development. Disease-modifying therapy can decrease cognitive loss.[30] Cognitive deficits are not necessarily irreversible. They can occur during an acute relapse, then improve during recovery.[31] Glucocorticoid treatment can be associated with iatrogenic worsening of cognitive function, which then improves once steroids are stopped. Ongoing studies are evaluating medications used to improve memory in Alzheimer patients (such as donepezil, [Aricept]) in cognitively impaired MS patients. Table 8.6 outlines an approach to the problem of cognitive loss in MS.

Table 8.6 Approach to cognitive impairment in MS.

- Education
  - Make sure patients, caregivers, and families are aware that MS can produce cognitive problems
  - Educate on the implications and manifestations of cognitive problems
- Document and identify extent of problem
  - If cognitive impairment is suspected, obtain formal neurocognitive function testing to identify involved domains, and severity of the problem
- Treatment approach must be individualized
  - Family counseling
  - Occupational counseling, vocational reassessment
  - Teach coping/compensation strategies
  - Consider cognitive rehabilitation
  - Consider pharmacotherapy
    - Optimize disease-modifying therapy
    - Memory drugs developed for Alzheimer's disease

Depression

Although depression is clearly the major mood disorder seen in MS, patients may experience a number of psychiatric problems and diverse mood disturbances (Table 8.7).[32,33] Some degree of euphoria occurs in about 25% of patients, but is sustained in less than 10%. Euphoria is associated with poorer cognitive and neurological function, greater social disability, and more pronounced brain atrophy. No effective therapy is known. Panic disorder can occur in MS, and appears to respond to valproic acid (Depakote). MS is associated with increased risk of bipolar affective disorder. Its frequency is twofold greater than in the normal population. This may require appropriate psychiatric treatment. MS patients with a family history of bipolar disorder are at particular risk. Episodes can be precipitated by glucocorticoid therapy, as can episodes of psychosis. Psychosis in MS has been associated with lesions involving the temporal lobe on MRI scan. Psychosis may respond to the atypical antipsychotic drug clozapine, which is an antagonist for D1, D2, and D4 dopamine receptors, as well as serotonin receptors. Emotional regulation disorder (inappropriate laughter or crying) occurs in 12% of MS patients. This reflects a pseudobulbar palsy syndrome, and usually responds to treatment with tricyclic antidepressants.

Approximately 50% of MS patients will experience clinical depression.[34] Depression can be reactive, due to disease damage or immune related disturbances, due to treatment effects, or any combination of these factors. When a young person is told (s)he has an incurable neurological disease which is unpredictable and likely to result in disability, it is not surprising that (s)he might become depressed. Depression can also occur during clinical relapse, presumably a result of neurochemical and neurotransmitter changes from disruption of cell function and circuitry. In one study, MS patients with depression and anxiety problems had evidence of hypothalamic–pituitary–adrenal gland axis dysfunction, and failed to suppress cortisol with dexamethasone pretreatment.[35] These systems correlated with CNS inflammation, as manifested by CSF pleocytosis and brain MRI contrast lesion activity. In another study, successful treatment of

Table 8.7 Psychiatric problems and mood disturbances in MS.

- Depression (27–75%)
- Irritability
- Poor concentration
- Anxiety/panic disorder
- Bipolar affective disorder
- Euphoria
- Psychosis
- Emotional regulation disorder

depression was associated with suppression of interferon gamma production by peripheral blood mononuclear cells.[36]

Since the rate of suicide is increased in the MS population, it is critical to identify and treat depressed patients. Warning signs include:

1. feelings of hopelessness and despair
2. decreased interest and pleasure in activities
3. change in appetite and weight (increased or decreased)
4. sleep disturbance (increased or decreased)
5. psychomotor disturbances (retardation or hyperactivity)
6. fatigue, loss of energy
7. feelings of worthlessness and guilt
8. inability to concentrate or make decisions
9. recurrent thoughts of death or suicide.

In some reports, interferon β therapy has been associated with worsening of depression.[37–39] Most affected patients had a prior history of depression. Recent trials of interferon β, although not confirming this association, do routinely screen out markedly depressed/suicidal patients. Although a history of depression is not a contraindication to interferon β therapy, patients and physicians should be aware of this potential drug complication. Optimal treatment probably involves a combination of antidepressants and psychotherapy, but either modality alone may be sufficient. Pharmacotherapy may involve older tricyclic antidepressants (which inhibit multiple neurotransmitter uptake sites, block multiple neuroreceptors, and influence second messenger systems and membrane ion channels), monoamine oxidase inhibitors, selective serotonin reuptake inhibitors, and a group of atypical antidepressants (buproprion, venlafaxine, nefazodone, mirtazapine, and reboxetine). An approach to treatment of depression is outlined in Table 8.8.

Table 8.8 Treatment of depression in MS.

- Educate patient and family about warning signs
- Discuss the problem
- Consider psychotherapy
- Consider antidepressant therapy
- Monitor response to treatment at regular intervals

Spasticity

Spasticity can be defined as a state of increased muscle tone, most apparent during stretching of muscles. It may occur during exercise, positional transfer, or fixed position. Spasticity indicates upper motor neuron/corticospinal tract dysfunction. Approximately 38% of patients complain of mild spasticity, while 32% complain of moderate to severe spasticity.[1] It is particularly frequent in progressive MS patients, who usually show spinal cord involvement. Spasticity may be so severe as to limit the ability to bend a joint or move legs apart. Although spasticity is most often due to lesions within the spinal cord, cerebral lesions can also produce increase in muscle tone.

Spasticity manifests as hyperreflexia, clonus, extensor plantar response, increased resistance to passive movement, flexor or extensor spasms, hyperextension, and exaggerated withdrawal response. It is often associated with slowed movement and weakness. Spasticity can be phasic (consisting of flexor or extensor spasms) or tonic (constant stiffness). More than half of all MS patients will experience spasticity, with legs more often involved than arms. In primary progressive MS, spasticity at onset of the disease (especially when it is bilateral) has a poorer prognosis.[40]

Acute worsening of spasticity is common during clinical relapse. Worsening can also be triggered by noxious stimuli such as urinary tract infection, full bladder or full bowel, or infected decubitus skin lesion.[41] Increased tone in an extremity is often brought on by specific positioning of a joint, such as bending a knee at a certain angle. It is usually most prominent in the morning, when the patient has been immobile overnight. Extensor spasms involve exaggerated extensor tone. These spasms may be quite painful, occur most often either at night in bed or on first getting up in the morning, and are most often seen in progressive MS. Flexor spasms involve exaggerated flexor tone. They are also often quite painful, and are typically seen in the later stages of the disease. Most of the consequences of spasticity are negative. Spasticity causes pain, poor posture, limited mobility, and can lead to contractures, skin breakdown, and infection. It disrupts sleep, interferes with activities of daily living and daily hygiene. It leads to social isolation and decreased quality of life. At the same time, it can also have a positive effect by enhancing the ability to walk, stand, and transfer in patients with very weak muscles.

The pathophysiology of spasticity involves dysfunction of multiple components of the motor system, including alpha and gamma motorneurons, descending monosynaptic and polysynaptic spinal pathways (these are the vestibulospinal, reticulospinal, monaminergic raphe serotonin and locus ceruleus norepinephrine tracts), interneurons (Ia, II and Ib), muscle spindles, and golgi tendon organs. Descending motor pathways can sprout to form new synapses on spinal neurons, leading to denervation supersensitivity. Alpha and gamma motor neurons, as well as Ia interneurons, become hyperexcitable. There may be decreased presynaptic inhibition, decreased recurrent (Renshaw cell) inhibition, decreased autogenic Ib afferent inhibition, and decreased reciprocal Ia afferent inhibition.

Interferon β can transiently worsen pre-existing spasticity, especially in temperature sensitive individuals. There may be two distinct mechanisms. During the first 12 weeks of therapy, increased spasticity can occur within

3–24 hours of injection. It typically lasts hours to days, and often occurs in the setting of flu-like symptoms. This can be treated with nonsteroidal anti-inflammatory agents or antispasticity agents. Spasticity can also increase in primary progressive patients who are on treatment for at least 2 months.[42] It lasts throughout treatment, but typically improves several months after interferon β is stopped.

Spasticity can be quantified by the use of a rating system such as the Ashworth scale (Table 8.9).[43] This can be used to provide a more quantitative treatment response for a given muscle group.

The treatment of spasticity involves identification and management of any triggering factors, physical strategies, pharmacotherapy, and in severe refractory cases surgical therapy (Table 8.10). Glucocorticoids often improve spasticity, but it is usually only temporary. In the past the usual approach has been to start with a single agent, push it to toxicity, and then switch to a second agent. However, a combination of low dose baclofen plus tizanidine may work better than either drug alone. In general, medical and physical therapy options are optimized before considering surgical intervention.

A key feature in the treatment of spasticity involves an effective physiotherapy program (Table 8.11). The goals of physiotherapy are to avoid secondary complications of pressure sores, prevent or treat contractures, decrease hypertonia, improve posture, develop or improve useful autonomous movements, and select appropriate supportive aides.

Pharmacotherapy for spasticity is outlined in Table 8.12.[44] These drugs have different mechanisms of action. Baclofen, tizanidine, and benzodiazepines all increase presynaptic inhibition of group I afferents. Tizanidine also decreases activity of excitatory interneurons, while dantrolene decreases muscle contractility.

Baclofen is a gamma-aminobutyric acid (GABA)-b agonist with pre- and postsynaptic actions. This receptor is particularly prominent in the spinal cord. It couples to calcium and potassium channels, and hyperpolarizes the presynaptic membrane. Baclofen acts on both monosynaptic and polysynaptic pathways. The drug has a half life of 3–4 hours, shows poor CNS penetration, is partially metabolized in the liver (about 15%), and is excreted in the urine. It comes in 10 and 20 mg tablets. The typical dosing

Table 8.9 Ashworth scale to evaluate spasticity.

Grade	Interpretation
0	No increase in tone
1	Slight increase in tone (catch during flexion–extension)
2	More marked increase in tone, but limb easily moved
3	Considerable increase in tone, passive movement difficult
4	Limb rigid, no passive mobilization

Table 8.10 Treatment of MS spasticity.

- Identify and correct/treat any precipitating factor
  - Infection
  - Relapse
  - Positioning
  - Constipation
  - Bedsore/decubitus
- Correct comorbidity factors
  - Physical deconditioning
  - Pain
  - Fatigue
- Physiotherapy program
  - Institute regular stretching and exercise programs
  - Heat or cold applications can be used to loosen muscles
  - Stretching/range of motion exercises carried out for at least 10–20 minutes
- Pharmacotherapy program
  - Start first line oral medications
    - Baclofen
    - Tizanidine
    - Combination
  - Try monotherapy combination
  - Use second line oral medications as needed
    - Benzodiazepines
    - Gabapentin
    - Dantrolene
    - Others
- Consider nonoral/surgical options
  - Intrathecal baclofen pump
  - Botox injections
  - Ablative surgery (rarely needed)

Table 8.11 Physiotherapy program for treatment of MS spasticity.

- Stretching
- Passive range of motion exercises
- Massage
- Proper positioning and posture
- Avoid positions that elicit clonus and spasms
- Appropriate splinting
- Application of cold packs/warm heat to relax muscles
- Transcutaneous electrical nerve stimulation (TENS)
- Appropriate use of accessory devices

range is 5 mg to 160 mg (or higher as tolerated), divided over a three or four times a day schedule. Baclofen should never be abruptly withdrawn, since discontinuation can be associated with seizures, hallucinations, and a marked rebound in spasticity. Side effects include muscle weakness, fatigue, drowsiness, nausea, dizziness, and ataxia. Baclofen lowers the seizure threshold, and can potentiate the effect of antihypertensives.

Table 8.12 Pharmacotherapy for MS spasticity.

- Primary drugs
  - Baclofen (Lioresal)
  - Tizanidine (Zanaflex)
- Secondary drugs
  - Benzodiazepines
    - Diazepam (Valium)
    - Clonazepam (Klonopin)
  - Gabapentin (Neurontin)
- Tertiary drugs
  - Botulinum toxin (Botox)
  - Clonidine (Catapres)
  - Dantrolene (Dantrium)
  - Threonine
  - Other agents
    - Cannabinoids
    - Phenothiazines
    - Opioids
    - Glucocorticoids
    - Cyproheptadine

Tizanidine is an imidazole derivative, and a centrally acting alpha$_2$-adrenergic agonist. It acts on both spinal and supraspinal receptor sites. Tizanidine inhibits release of excitatory amino acids from spinal interneurons. Its major effect is on presynaptic spinal cord activity, but it also inhibits postsynaptic excitation, increases postsynaptic inhibition, and inhibits alpha motor neurons. There is a modest supraspinal effect, at the level of the locus ceruleus. The half life is 2–4 (average 2.5) hours. Tizanidine shows an absorption rate of 53–66%. The drug is metabolized by liver microsomal enzymes, and is excreted in the urine (53–66% of drug) and feces (19–23% of drug). Tizanidine comes in 2 mg and 4 mg tablets. It is dosed in the 2–36 mg range, divided over a three times a day schedule. Tizanidine can cause hypotension, so that a test dose should be given. The dose is slowly titrated upwards over 2–4 weeks. Side effects include dry mouth, somnolence and drowsiness (in 24–48% of patients), dizziness (10–19%), and hepatoxicity (liver transaminases increase in 5–7% of patients).[45] Muscle weakness (18–48%) is less common than with baclofen.

Benzodiazepines include long acting and short acting agents which bind within brainstem and spinal cord. These drugs both potentiate a presynaptic GABA effect, but also have a postsynaptic action. Clonazepam comes in 0.5, 1, and 2 mg tablets. Typical dosing ranges from 0.5 to 10 mg daily, given over a three or four times a day schedule. Diazepam binds to the GABA-a receptor, increases chloride conductance, increases presynaptic inhibition, and acts to enhance inhibition at a spinal cord level. The dosing range is 2 mg to 60 mg, divided typically three or four times a day. This is despite its very long half life of 20–80 hours. After oral intake, levels peak at 1 hour. Diazepam is 98% protein bound, and metabolized by the liver. Side effects include sedation, cognitive blunting, dependence, weakness, GI problems, depression, and ataxia. Abrupt withdrawal of diazepam has precipitated seizures, so that it is typically tapered.

Gabapentin is a GABA analog. The drug binds at distinct GABA receptors, rather than the a or b receptor. Levels peak 2–3 hours after an oral dose. Gabapentin is excreted unchanged in the urine. The typical dosing range is 300–3600 mg a day, divided over a three times a day schedule. Anecedotal data suggests the antispasticity effect is not seen under 1200 mg four times a day.[46] Side effects include somolence, dizzinesss, ataxia, and tremor.

Clonidine is a centrally acting alpha$_2$-adrenergic receptor agonist. It is generally used as an add-on agent for spasticity, rather than as monotherapy. It comes in 0.1 mg tablets, and an 0.1 and 0.2 mg patch that is typically used weekly. Side effects include bradycardia, hypotension, dry mouth, drowsiness, constipation, dizziness, and depression.

Dantrolene sodium is a hydantoin derivative. It has a direct effect on muscle, resulting in decreased release of calcium from sarcoplasmic reticulum. As a result, there is a decrease in excitation contraction coupling. Dantrolene affects fast twitch and extrafusal fibers. It comes in 25, 50, and 100 mg tablets, with the typical dosing range of 25–400 mg daily. The drug half life is 15 hours, with peak levels 3–6 hours after an oral dose. Dantrolene is metabolized in the liver. Side effects include weakness, drowsiness, and diarrhea. Hepatotoxocity is the major concern, particularly in women over 30 who use the drug chronically. Prior liver damage puts patients at increased risk, so that liver enzymes should be measured prior to as well as during therapy.

Cannabinoids act on the CB1 cannabinoid receptor in the CNS, to inhibit cyclic AMP and voltage dependent calcium channels. This has an antispastic effect. Synthetic cannabinoids are being evaluated for symptom management of MS spasticity, as well as tremor, pain, and bladder disturbances.

Botulinum toxin blocks presynaptic acetycholine release, in effect producing a chemical denervation. There are A through G toxins, although toxin A and more recently B are the ones in clinical use. Botulinum toxin injection is useful when there is spasticity in a "functional unit", such as spasticity/spasms localized to the adductor muscles.[47] Typically 500–1000 units of toxin are injected into the muscle. Focal paralysis begins at 24–72 hours, peaks at 24–72 hours, and lasts 12–16 weeks. The treatment is impractical when spasticity affects multiple muscles.

With regard to nonoral therapy for spasticity, a number of surgical procedures have been used.[48] The major treatment has been the intrathecal

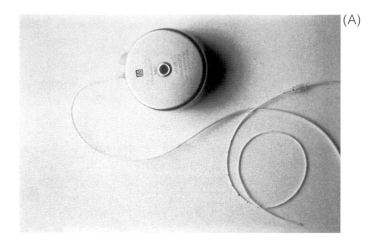

(A)

(B)

(C)

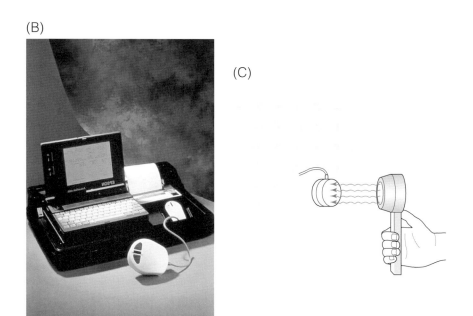

Figure 8.3
An effective treatment for refractory spasticity is the delivery of intrathecal
baclofen via a pump (A) that is surgically implanted under the abdominal skin.
The pump is programmed with a computer (B) and dosage instructions are
delivered through a radiofrequency signal (C). (Courtesy of Medtronic)

baclofen pump. Patients undergo a presurgical test dosing which involves admission to the hospital for lumbar puncture and installation of 50–100 µg baclofen. This should produce marked decrease in tone which lasts hours. This trial is done to assure a patient response, before proceeding to more invasive surgery. Intrathecal baclofen is delivered by a surgically implanted, programmable pump (Figure 8.3 A,B,C). Drug is infused into the CSF at around L3–4. The advantages of this delivery system are that it uses a much smaller dose of baclofen, instills it directly into the CNS compartment, and has much less systemic side effects. The dose can actually be varied over a 24-hour period, with a different amount of baclofen infused, for example, overnight during sleep. The maintenance dose of intrathecal baclofen ranges from 300 to 800 µg over a 24-hour period. The pump is placed subcutaneously in the anterior abdominal region, and is refilled approximately every 6–12 weeks percutaneously. Liquid baclofen is stable for at least 3 months. The pump must be replaced after several years.

Pain and sensory disturbances

Pain is a common positive sensory symptom of MS. Ultimately up to 75% of MS patients experience pain at some point in their illness, although it is unusual as an early feature.[49] The one exception is trigeminal neuralgia. For a minority of patients pain is their major MS complaint. It can be acute or chronic. One way to categorize MS pain is whether it is due to the MS disease process (primary), is a secondary MS complication, or is due to an unrelated coincidental condition (Table 8.13).

The generation of neuropathic pain is not understood, but may involve spontaneous impulses due to disturbed sodium channel expression. Nerve impulses depend upon these channels, and after axon injury sodium channel genes are both activated and inactivated. Neuropathic pain includes trigeminal neuralgia, painful tonic spasms, continuous dysesthetic pain, and acute radicular pain. Trigeminal neuralgia is a striking syndrome of brief, shock-like pain, typically in the distribution of V2 or V3, which can occur spontaneously or with cutaneous trigger zones. Movement, touch, or even a gust of wind can generate pain. Most cases of trigeminal neuralgia are unrelated to MS and occur in patients over age 50. Trigeminal neuralgia in a young person should always raise the possibility of MS, since this syndrome occurs in almost 2% of all patients. Trigeminal neuralgia is bilateral in close to 20% of cases. It is treated with anticonvulsants such as carbamazepine (Tegretol), phenytoin (Dilantin), clonazepam (Klonopin), gabapentin (Neurontin), or lamotrigine (Lamictal). Gabapentin and lamotrigine are newer anticonvulsants that work by inhibiting the release of glutamate through blockade of voltage dependent sodium channels. Combination therapy with low dose gabapentin (800–850 mg every day), plus carbamazepine (400 mg) or lamotrigine (150 mg), may be better

Table 8.13 MS pain syndromes.

Primary Pain Syndrome
• Acute neuropathic pain
  – Neuralgias
  – Lhermitte
  – Dysesthesias
• Chronic neuropathic pain
  – Central pain syndrome
  – Burning causalgia-like pain
  – Optic neuritis related chronic photophobia
• Acute inflammatory process pain
• Secondary pain syndromes
  – Spasticity related
  – Musculoskeletal (back, joints)
  – Skin breakdown, pressure points
  – Bladder spasms
  – Vertebral compression
• Unrelated pain syndromes
  – Headache
  – Malignancy
  – Trauma
  – Musculoskeletal (back, joints)

tolerated than high dose monotherapy. Baclofen and misoprosil have also been used. Surgical therapies include neurolytic procedures. Percutaneous controlled radiofrequency rhizotomy is the most commonly used technique. Glycerol rhizolysis, percutaneous microcompression, alcoholic neurolysis, and external beam gamma knife radiosurgery have also been used.[50]

Painful tonic spasms are almost MS specific. They occur in 10–20% of patients. Spasms last for less than 2 minutes, are extremely painful, and affect a very focal region. They can be triggered by movement or sensory input. Attacks generally occur repetitively over several weeks. Tonic spasms are probably due to a corticospinal tract lesion. They respond well to antiseizure medication.

Continuous dysesthetic pain is a syndrome of burning pain involving most often one or both legs. It is the most common MS neuropathic pain syndrome, and can be thought of as a central pain syndrome. Patients have proprioceptive (large fiber) loss, and to a lesser degree pain and temperature loss. Treatment includes tricyclic antidepressants and anticonvulsants (carbamazepine, gabapentin, lamotrigine).

The final neuropathic pain syndrome, acute radicular pain, is unusual in MS. It can occur as a presenting complaint, following trauma, or as a spontaneous problem.

Acute inflammation is an integral component of the MS disease process, particularly in the early years. Inflammation can result in pain, most likely due to activation of dural nociceptors. The best example is optic neuritis, which regularly involves pain on eye movement. This pain responds nicely to glucocorticoids.

Secondary disease complications result in pain problems. The best example is spasticity, which invariably causes some degree of muscle pain. Manifestations include muscle spasms and cramps. Lower extremities are most commonly affected. The treatment of spasticity related pain involves physiotherapy as well as standard antispasticity agents. Cannabinoids may also help spasticity related pain.

Nonspecific pain syndromes can also occur in MS patients. Headache appears to be more common in MS than the general population, and may occur with acute relapses. There is no characteristic MS headache however, and both vascular and muscle contraction headaches are seen particularly in young patients. Musculoskeletal back pain also occurs in MS patients. This can be a combination of degenerative changes along facet joints, foramina, and disk disease, as well as myofacial pain due to spasticity and a disease relapse. In patients with back pain the possibility of urinary tract or kidney infection should be considered. For MS patients who have received frequent glucocorticoids, osteoporosis and vertebral collapse should be considered.

Optimal treatment of pain depends on the underlying cause and syndrome (Tables 8.14,15). Pain due to spasticity, related problems, disuse, and poor posture should be treated with aggressive physical therapy and antispasticity regimens. Pain due to inflammatory disease activity will respond to anti-inflammatory/glucocorticoid therapy and should be self limited. Pain due to neurological damage (neuropathic pain) can be paroxysmal or chronic. Paroxysmal pain generally responds well to anticonvulsants. Chronic neuropathic pain may be the most difficult to treat, but is often blunted by tricyclic antidepressants or anticonvulsants. Pain in comorbid symptoms can make other symptoms such as fatigue and depression worse, and makes them more refractory to therapy. Therefore it is important to treat pain in MS aggressively and effectively. It should be minimized if it cannot be totally removed.

Paroxysmal attacks

Paroxysmal symptoms probably represent ephaptic synaptic nerve conduction along damaged nerve pathways. There are a variety of brief, stereotypic symptoms which occur repeatedly many times a day (Table 8.16).[51] Painful tonic spasms would be one manifestation of this symptom. Although paroxysmal attacks do not reflect true seizure activity, they usually respond well to anticonvulsant therapy. Low dose carbamazepine,

Table 8.14 Treatment of MS pain syndromes.

Syndrome	Therapy

Acute neuralgia	Anticonvulsants
	    Carbamazepine (100–1600 mg)
	    Phenyntoin (100–500 mg)
	    Gabapentin (100–3600 mg)
	    Lamotrigine (100 mg)
	Tricyclic antidepressants (25–150 mg)
	Baclofen (10–120 mg)
	Glucocorticoids (60–100 mg+)

Chronic neuropathic pain	Surgical procedures
	    Rhizotomy/rhizolysis
	    Microcompression
	    Radiosurgery
	Tricyclic antidepressants
	Anticonvulsants

Acute inflammatory process pain	Glucocorticoids/anti-inflammatory agents
Secondary pain syndromes	Control spasticity and spasms Improve posture; muscle strengthening Prophylactic skin care Nonsteroidal anti-inflammatory agents Local ice/heat packs Massage/ultrasound therapy Range of motion stretching exercises Injection therapy (trigger point, facet joint)
Unrelated pain syndromes	Appropriate diagnosis followed by symptomatic management

Table 8.15 Surgical treatments for MS pain.

- Intrathecal phenol
- Cordectomy
- Dorsal column stimulation
- Dorsal root section/entry zone lesion
- Myclotomy

phenytoin, and baclofen can be very effective. An acute vestibular syndrome can occur, characterized by nausea, vomiting, vertigo, and postular instability. Persistent central nausea has responded to ondansetron (Zofran), presumably by blockade at the level of the vomiting center.

Table 8.16 Paroxysmal MS symptoms.

- Paroxysmal attacks
  - Brief repetitive episodes (hemiparesis, ataxia, dysarthria, dystonia, painful tonic spasms, vertigo) loss of tone, kinesogenic choroethetosis
- Sensory phenomenon
  - Lhermittes
  - Paresthesias
  - Neuralgia
- Facial movements
  - Myokymia
  - Hemifacial spasm
- Segmental myoclonus
- Hiccups

Tremor

Some degree of tremor, particularly affecting the arms, is found in almost 60% of MS patients.[52] This action (postural-intention) tremor is believed to reflect brainstem-cerebellar circuitry lesions, and is one of the most difficult to treat MS symptoms. It indicates more severe disease and a worse prognosis, and is incapacitating in 10% of patients. There is no satisfactory therapy, although a variety of drugs and assistive devices have been used with some benefit (Table 8.17). Drugs are generally tried on a trial and error basis, since a given drug may promote a modest benefit. Ondansetron is a very expensive anti-nausea medication. It is a 5-hydroxytryptamine receptor antagonist. Ondansetron has been reported to benefit cerebellar tremor. Combined treatment with gabapentin and lamotrigine has also been reported to

Table 8.17 Symptomatic treatment for tremor.

- Identify type of tremor, body parts involved, any triggering factors
- Identify helpful assistive devices, braces, support
  - Therapy evaluation
- Consider trials of medicines
  - Propranolol
  - Mysoline
  - Clonazepam
  - Gabapentin
  - Lamotrigine
  - Carbamazepine
  - Phenytoin
  - Isoniazid
  - Ondansetron

have some benefit. Surgical therapies which have been tried for tremor include both ablative and stimulation techniques. Stereotactic neurostimulation of the ventral intermediate thalamic nucleus is being used to treat essential and Parkinsonian tremors, and there are reports of benefit in some patients.

Bowel and bladder

Bowel and bladder dysfunction, also considered sphincter disturbances, often go together. They are not usually prominent symptoms early in the MS disease course, but over time most patients will experience problems. Although most bowel and bladder problems reflect spinal cord lesions, so that patients often have associated impaired walking ability, cerebral lesions can also produce sphincter disturbances. There are three types of neurogenic bladder (Table 8.18).[53] Detrusor hyperreflexia, the most common form of neurogenic MS bladder, involves spontaneous inappropriate contractions of the bladder muscle. Patients experience marked frequency and urgency. Detrusor sphincter dyssynergia means that when the bladder detrusor muscle contracts there is paradoxic contraction of the sphincter as well, so that the urine cannot be expelled properly. Normally the sphincter muscle relaxes to allow urination (Figure 8.4). The least common form of neurogenic bladder, detruser hyporeflexia, involves failure of the detrusor muscle to contract, resulting in urinary retention. Bladder dysfunction occurs in 50–80% of patients, and typically parallels severity of other symptoms, particularly motor system problems.[54] The severity of bladder dysfunction is unrelated to disease duration. Problems are disruptive rather than life threatening, and often fluctuate over time. General measures can be useful to treat a mild neurogenic bladder (Table 8.19). Detrusor hyperreflexia generally responds to anticholinergics, although they can produce bothersome side effects of dry mouth, blurred vision,

Table 8.18 Neurogenic bladder in MS.

- Detrusor hyperreflexia (50–90%; spastic bladder, failure to store)
    - Symptoms of urgency, frequency, incontinence, nocturia
    - Postvoid residual normal (< 100 cc)
- Detrusor sphincter dyssynergia (25–40%; combined dysfunction)
    - Symptoms of dribbling, incontinence, incomplete emptying, double voiding, urgency, hesitancy
    - Postvoid residual may be normal (< 100 cc) or increased (> 100 cc)
- Detrusor hyporeflexia (20%; flacid bladder, failure to empty)
    - Symptoms of incomplete emptying, urgency, frequency, hesitancy, double voiding
    - Postvoid residual increased (> 100 cc)

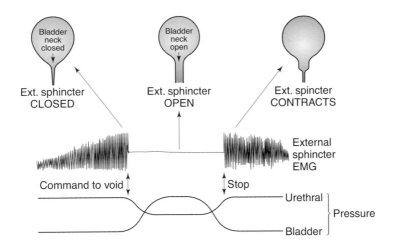

Figure 8.4
Bladder and external sphincter muscles must be synchronized to allow successful voiding.

and tachycardia. Nocturia can respond to limitation of fluids at night-time, use of an anticholinergic at night, or use of the nasal spray desmopressin acetate (DDAVP), a synthetic diuretic hormone analog.[55] Potential side effects of this spray include hypertension and edema.

Urinary tract infections can worsen bladder symptoms, and may also be a trigger for disease flareups. Urine may be screened for infection by dipstick (particularly the leukocyte esterase) or a microscopic urinalysis.[56] Uncomplicated infections are treated for 3–7 days, while recurrent infections or those associated with fever should be treated for 7–14 days. However, in patients with an indwelling catheter who are symptom free (no fever, flank pain, or change in health status), infection does not necessarily need to be treated. Bacteriuria can reflect simple colonization. In any female patient who has three or more urinary tract infections within a year, and probably in any male patient with a single urinary tract infection, imaging studies (bladder ultrasound, intravenous urogram) are indicated to rule out structural pathology. Tips to prevent urinary tract infections are outlined in Table 8.20.

Intermittent catheterization is generally necessary when the bladder does not fully empty, since stagnant urine predisposes to infection. Catheterization is much more difficult for women than men. Before prescribing catheterization, it is important to make sure that it is acceptable to the patient.[56] It also has to be feasible. Patients with limited manual dexterity, cognitive or visual impairment, spasticity, or marked fatigue may have difficulty. There may need to be assistance, including access to accessible restrooms.

Table 8.19 Treatment of neurogenic bladder.

General measures
- Use of bedside commode or urinal
- Schedule fluid intake
- Try to arrange timed voiding
- Establish emptying techniques every three hours initially
  - Tapping over suprapubic region
  - Crede manuever
  - Straining to empty bladder
- Intermittent catherization every 4–6 hours
  - To maintain < 400 cc in bladder
- Use of pads and special undergarments as needed

Detrusor hyperreflexia (spastic bladder)
- Anticholinergics if postvoid residual <100 cc (typically <10 cc)
  - Oxybutynin (Ditropan, Ditropan XL)
  - Tolterodine (Detrol, Detrol LA)
  - Imipramine (Tofranil)
  - Hyoscyamine (Levsin, Cytospaz),
  - Propantheline (Probanthine)
- Vasopressin anolog (DDAVP nasal spray)
- Intravesical capsacin
- Additional techniques
  - Scheduled fluid intake
  - Scheduled/prompted voiding
  - Avoidance of caffeine, alcohol, aspartame
  - Pelvic floor exercises
  - Other behavioral modifications
- Failure to respond, or postvoid residual >100 cc
  - Proceed to urodynamics and imaging studies

Detrusor sphincter dyssynergia
- Regular attempts to void (light tapping)
- Antispasticity agents
  - Baclofen
  - Tizanidine
  - Benzodiazepines
- Alpha-adrenergic blocking agents
  - Doxazosin (Cardura)
  - Phenoxybenzamine (Dibenzyline)
  - Prazosin (Minipres)
  - Clonidine (Catapres)
  - Terazosin (Hytrin)
- Alpha$_2$-agonist
  - Clonidine
- Anticholinergic agents with intermittent catheterization

Detrusor hyporeflexia (flaccid bladder)
- Intermittent catheterization
- Alpha blocker plus emptying techniques
- Cholinergic agents (bethanechol, Urecholine) plus emptying techniques

Table 8.20 Tips to prevent urinary tract infection.

- Be aware of the signs of infection (pain, odor, cloudy urine, change in bladder status)
- Try to completely empty bladder
- Drink enough fluids (6–8 glasses)
- Increase urine acidity (Vitamin C)
- Women should wipe front to back when going to the bathroom
- Change indwelling catheters monthly

Table 8.21 Management of bowel problems in MS.

General measures
- Establish regular bowel regimen
  - Scheduled evacuation times
- Assure adequate daily dietary fiber (15 g) daily
  - High fiber foods (fruits, vegetables, grains)
  - Supplements (psyllium, metamucil)
  - Avoid rice, cheese; excess protein
- Assure adequate daily hydration (1.5–2 liters)

Constipation
- Start by cleaning out the bowel
- Use dietary triggers (100% bran, fruit and apple juice, other fluids/foods)
- Oral medications
  - Bulk forming agents
  - Stool softeners (docusate sodium, docusate/casanthranol)
  - Smooth muscle stimulants (senna) 6–8 hours before evacuation
  - Mild laxatives
- Local stimulant
  - Suppositories (Bisacodil, glycerin)
  - Digital stimulation
- Local evacuants
  - Ther-evac mini enema, fleet enema
- Systemic stimulants
  - Magnesium citrate
- Biofeedback retraining

Fecal incontinence
- Bowel training regimen/programmed evacuation times
  - Avoid chronically distended rectum
- Appropriate diet
- Suppositories to evacuate rectum
- Anticholinergic medications
- Surgical maneuvers
  - Rectal bag
  - Artificial sphincter

Diarrhea
- Monitor diet, weight, electrolytes
- Skin care
- Replace fluid loss
- Medications to decrease GI mobility (antidiarrheals)
- Bulk forming supplements
- Biofeedback retraining

Bowel dysfunction may occur with or without bladder problems. It is reported in 41–68% of patients. The most common problem is with elimination (constipation), but there can also be problems with storage (diarrhea, fecal incontinence), and both problems may coexist in the same patient. Several conditions contribute to MS bowel dysfunction. Constipation may reflect slow colonic transit time, poor mobility, abnormal rectal function, pelvic floor dysfunction, use of anticholinergics/muscle relaxants, intussusception, and decreased fluid intake. Fecal incontinence can reflect decreased rectal filling sensation, poor sphincter and pelvic floor contraction, decreased rectal compliance, obstetric injury, and a weak rectal sphincter. The patient's diet may be inadequate, and a neurogenic bowel results in decreased normal bowel motility after eating. An approach to treating MS bowel problems is outlined in Table 8.21. Behavioral techniques include counseling, education, and biofeedback.

Sexual dysfunction

Sexual dysfunction is unusual as an early symptom in MS, but ultimately up to 91% of men and 72% of women report sexual problems (Table 8.22).[53] They are multifactorial, and include psychologic as well as physiologic dysfunction.[57] This is an important symptom, which affects marital relationships in up to 71% of cases.[58] Sexual dysfunction may be a primary symptom or a secondary symptom (difficulty with positioning due to spasticity; presence of a catheter). It can also be iatrogenic, a side effect of medication used to treat MS symptoms. This is particularly true for serotonin reuptake inhibitors. Sexual dysfunction can relate to lesions in the spinal cord lateral columns that synapse on autonomic nervous system neurons in the lower thoracic and upper lumbar cord, lesions that affect sacral parasympathetic as well as thoracolumbar sympathetic outflow, and higher (cortical) lesions. Most sexual dysfunction problems appear to relate to suprasacral lesions.[59-61] Treatment of sexual dysfunction requires a multifactorial approach (Table 8.23). Associated bladder dysfunction should be carefully assessed. Sildenafil citrate (Viagra) has been particularly helpful for erectile dysfunction.[62] This is a phosphodiesterase type 5 inhibitor which is taken 1 hour before intercourse to facilitate an erection. Arousal is necessary however. The response rate is about 70%. There are potential drug interactions with macrolide antibiotics imetidine and oral antifungal agents. Sildenafil should not be used in patients with significant coronary artery disease. Side effects occur in 6–18% of patients, and include dyspepsia, flushing, nasal congestion, and headache.

Table 8.22 Sexual dysfunction in MS.

- Anorgasmia
- Decreased libido
- Erectile dysfunction
- Lubrication problems
- Decreased sensation
- Problems with ejaculation
- Decreased satisfaction
- Absent sexual activity
- Fatigued performance
- Decreased arousal

Table 8.23 Treatment of sexual dysfunction in MS.

General measures
- Frank discussion with patient and sex partner to identify problems
- Sexual counseling on alternative methods to penetration
  - Cuddling, touching, oral stimulation
- Treatment of complicating factors such as spasticity, pain, depression, fatigue, bowel/bladder problems
- Change in sexual positioning

Women
- Lubrication/moisturizer
- Use of vibrators and sex toys

Men
- Sildenafil citrate (Viagra)
- Injection of papaverine (Pavabid)
- Prostaglandin E_1 (alprostadil) insertion or injection
  - Muse system
  - Caverject
- Vacuum pumps
- Yohimbine
- Penile prosthesis
  - Inflatable
  - Semirigid (malleable)

Other symptoms

Weakness is present in about 80% of MS patients, and is almost invariable in progressive MS. The most common problem is bilateral asymmetric leg weakness (paraparesis), followed by weakness of one leg, and then weakness of an arm and leg (hemiparesis). Isolated weakness of one arm is unusual. Weakness in MS can be produced by disruption of descending supraspinal input to spinal premotor interneurons and neurons, by damage to spinal pathways, and as an indirect consequence of muscle, tendon and joint changes in patient with longstanding limitations in mobility. Treatment involves a regular exercise program to strengthen muscles, combined with cardiovascular conditioning, and appropriate use of assistive devices. Functional electrical stimulation is being studied.

Some degree of ataxia occurs in up to 75% of MS patients, often accompanied by tremor. Ataxia has as profound an effect on motor coordination as does weakness. Treatment involves patient education, rehabilitative strategies, assistive devices, and the same medications used to treat tremor.

Visual disturbances can result from optic neuritis as well as abnormal eye movements. Optic neuritis can lead to permanent impaired vision, color vision loss, or scotomatous field defect. Sometimes visual deficits are only noted with exercise or heat (Uthoff's syndrome). In later more severe MS occasionally vision loss can be progressive. Eye movement abnormalities can produce diplopia, nystagmus, and oscillopsia. Treatment approaches include specific drugs (baclofen, clonazepam, memantine, scopolamine, gabapentin, isoniazid, propranolol). Both gabapentin, and the glutamate receptor antagonist memantine, have been reported to benefit oscillopsia. Injection of botulinum toxin into discrete extraocular muscles has been used, and prisms may be helpful to treat both diplopia and nystagmus.

Dysphagia is uncommon in MS, but it is potentially life threatening. MS can affect the orolingual and oropharyngeal phases of deglutition secondary to muscle weakness, apraxia, or pseudobulbar palsy syndrome. Upper motor neuron dysphagia, as well as a decreased swallowing reflex, produces more problems with liquids, while defective tongue manipulation produces more problems with solids. Signs of dysphagia are choking and coughing. MS patients with dysphagia should avoid very dry foods and large pieces of food. A speech and language pathology consultation as well as a modified barium swallow study to evaluate food bolus manipulation and deglutition, can be helpful in MS patients with dysphagia. Therapeutic maneuvers include chin tuck when swallowing, turning the head to the weak side to help close the vocal cords, changing the consistency of food and liquid intake, and changing the swallow sequence ("swallow–cough–swallow" technique).

The most common speech problem in MS is dysarthria. Pseudobulbar palsy usually produces some degree of hypernasality. When severe it can result in speech apraxia or even anarthria. Treatment of speech problems involves behavioral modification: slower speech to improve pronunciation syllable by syllable. Orolingual exercises can improve mouth and tongue motor control. Patients can be taught to vary pitch, volume, and duration of syllables. In severe speech problems, alternative communication techniques may be needed. They can range from the use of paper and pencil to computerized communication boards.

Pressure ulcers affect severely disabled MS patients due to their inability to walk, motor paralysis, sensory deficits, cognitive loss, bladder and bowel incontinence, and malnutrition. Ulcers result from combinations of pressure, shearing forces, and moisture. Preventive measures include frequent changes in position, appropriate transfer, pressure relieving exercises, use of specialized mattresses and pressure relief and redistribution cushions, good fluid intake, high calorie protein-rich diets, and regular skin examination.

Aids for ambulation

Mobility can be impaired by weakness, spasticity, incoordination, proprioceptive deficits, or visual impairment. Appropriate use of assistive devices can improve ambulation and safety, and avoid falls. Canes include straight (standard) canes, palm canes, narrow-base quad canes, or wide base quad canes. They are used on the side contralateral to the weak limb. Crutches can be axillary or nonaxillary (Lofstrand crutches, Canadian crutches). Walkers may be without wheels (regular), with front wheels (rolling walker), or made for use with one hand (hemiwalker). The larger the device the more stable it is, but the less speed it allows. Walking assistive devices relieve weight bearing by 20–25%, axillary crutches by 80%, and nonaxillary crutches by 40–50%. Canes and Lofstrand crutches should be adjusted to allow 20–30° elbow flexion when they are in contact with the ground. This is not necessary for Canadian crutches, which keep the elbow extended. Walkers should be kept to 10–12 inches (25–30 cm) in front of the body. They are used with an erect posture, and with elbows flexed 15–20°.

Orthotics can be useful assistive devices to aid ambulation, but need frequent monitoring to reassess appropriateness. For patients with foot drop or spasticity, an ankle foot orthosis (AFO) brace can be helpful. Ideally it is lightweight, flexible, and specifically fitted, although patients can initially try out a prefabricated AFO off the shelf. An AFO offers mediolateral support for an unstable ankle. When that is not a factor, and correction of poor toe clearing is needed, a smaller AFO called a posterior leaf splint may be used. Lower limb orthoses must be comfortable, cosmetically acceptable, and easy to put on and remove. They should provide a good foot and leg angle, allow functional ambulation, avoid excessive pressure points, not compress the peroneal nerve, and not allow the knee to buckle.

Although a knee ankle foot orthosis (KAFO) is sometimes used in patients with poor ankle control and very weak quadriceps, it requires much more energy expenditure, is not as aesthetically pleasing, and is not tolerated by most MS patients. A possible substitute is a knee shell with or without an AFO.

Wheelchairs can be helpful for patients who are ambulatory but cannot walk long distances. Appropriate use of a wheelchair can allow patients to leave their home and engage in social and recreational activities. It is important, however, to encourage ambulatory patients to use a wheelchair only when truly needed. Manual wheelchairs should be easy to maneuver and not too bulky. The typical manual wheelchair weighs about 50 pounds (23 kg). Lightweight chairs range from 30 to 40 pounds (14–18 kg), while ultralight wheelchairs range from 20 to 25 pounds (9–11 kg). Front wheel wheelchairs are easier to maneuver and turn, but require more patient effort. Rear wheel wheelchairs are more commonly used in MS. Power assist wheels can be substituted for standard wheels so that pushing effect is enhanced by a wheel hub motor. Motorized scooters are useful in patients with impaired ambulation who are unable to propel a regular wheelchair or who become too tired. They can involve three or four wheels. Patients should be able to ambulate and maneuver, have reasonable trunkal control, and be able to swivel in and out of the wheelchair. Nonambulatory patients can use a more controllable motorized (electric) wheelchair, which can be directed by a single toggle switch requiring as little as one finger for control. Patients need to be able to sit, but are typically unable to maneuver. Any MS patient prescribed a wheelchair should be instructed in how to use it. Cognitively impaired patients may not do well with scooters or electric wheelchairs, and this should be a serious consideration before prescribing it.

Rehabilitation medicine

Rehabilitation medicine encompasses a number of areas, including use of assistive devices (Table 8.24). The goals of these rehabilitative techniques are to improve function, minimize loss of function, minimize or prevent secondary complications, achieve functional independence, reintegrate the patient into social and family situations, and assure efficient use of medical and community resources.[63] Rehabilitation medicine should facilitate impaired individuals to realize their optimal physical, mental, and social potential, to integrate them into an appropriate environment, and ultimately to improve their sense of well being. For the MS patient this generally involves an active and somewhat complex process of compensation rather than restoration. Working muscles need to be activated, while avoiding overload and conduction block.

Table 8.24 Rehabilitation medicine techniques.

- Physical therapy
- Occupational therapy
- Cognitive therapy
- Recreational therapy
- Vocational therapy
- Speech therapy
- Assistive devices
- Exercise program with meditative/mindful aspect (Tai Chi, Qi Gong)

Patient education and self management are critical to an effective rehabilitation program. It is important to understand the patient's perception of disability. Rehabilitative therapies for MS face a number of disease-specific complications. First, MS has a variable course and deficits are not fixed. Progressive patients gradually worsen, while relapsing patients can show dramatic and unpredictable fluctuations in disability. Second, the disabilities in this disease are complex. This requires one to prioritize, focus, and define success for the individual patient. Third, many patients have a variety of comorbid symptoms which impact on each other, and which may be differentially affected by a rehabilitation program. Ideally, there is an initial multidisciplinary assessment to identify the patient's perspective and circumstances, to design goal-oriented programs and evaluate achieved goals, and to evaluate the impact on the patient. Patients must be active participants. The complete rehabilitation therapy team involves the neurologist or pshychiatrist, physical therapist, occupational therapist, speech and language pathologist, recreational therapist, social worker, rehabilitation nurse, dietitian, neuropsychologist, and orthotic specialist. Recent studies document the benefits of exercise. An aerobic exercise program, 40 minutes three times a week, increases endurance, oxygen utilization, muscle strength, and sense of well being in MS patients.[64] It also improves depression, fatigue, and socialization. Patients improved with regard to bladder and bowel function, triglyceride level, and very low density lipoprotein levels. Intensive physical therapy programs can improve muscle strength and functional level. A general physical therapy program emphasizes ambulation, while occupational therapy emphasizes upper extremity hand function. Any exercise program for MS patients should incorporate cooling techniques, in order to allow maximal participation, by minimizing risk of conduction block.

Coping strategies to improve mindfulness of movement (Tai Chi, Qi Gong) have also been used to improve balance. They have been reported to improve a number of MS symptoms.

Summary

Symptomatic treatment is a cornerstone for optimal management of MS. Although symptoms may not be relieved entirely, they can be substantially improved through a multimodality approach combining appropriate education/awareness programs, lifestyle changes, rehabilitative strategies, pharmacotherapy, and surgical procedures. MS patients benefit from appropriate symptom management.

References

1. Goodin DS. Survey of multiple sclerosis in northern California. Northern California MS Study Group. Mult Scler 1999; 5:78–88.

2. Metz L. Multiple sclerosis: symptomatic therapies. Semin Neurol 1998; 18:389–395.

3. Krupp LB, Coyle PK, Doscher C, et al. Fatigue therapy in multiple sclerosis: results of a double-blind, randomized, parallel trial of amantadine, pemoline, and placebo. Neurology 1995; 45:1956–1961.

4. Schapiro RT. Symptom management in multiple sclerosis, 3rd edn. New York: Demos; 1998.

5. Multiple Sclerosis Council for Clinical Practice Guidelines. Fatigue and multiple sclerosis. Evidence-based management strategies for fatigue in multiple sclerosis. Paralyzed Veterans of America; 1998.

6. Comi G, Leocani L, Rossi P, Colombo B. Physiopathology and treatment of fatigue in multiple sclerosis. J Neurol 2001; 248:174–179.

7. Giovannoni G, Thompson AJ, Miller DH, Thompson EJ. Fatigue is not associated with raised inflammatory markers in multiple sclerosis. Neurology 2001; 57:676–681.

8. Sharma KR, Kent-Braun J, Mynhier MA, et al. Evidence of an abnormal intramuscular component of fatigue in multiple sclerosis. Muscle Nerve 1995; 18:1403–1411.

9. Sheean GL, Murray NM, Rothwell JC, et al. An electrophysiological study of the mechanism of fatigue in multiple sclerosis. Brain 1997; 120(Pt 2):299–315.

10. Kent-Braun JA, Sharma KR, Weiner MW, Miller RG. Effects of exercise on muscle activation and metabolism in multiple sclerosis. Muscle Nerve 1994; 17:1162–1169.

11. Roelcke U, Kappos L, Lechner-Scott J, et al. Reduced glucose metabolism in the frontal cortex and basal ganglia of multiple sclerosis patients with fatigue: a 18^F-fluorodeoxyglucose positron emission tomography study. Neurology 1997; 48:1566–1571.

12. Sandroni P, Walker C, Starr A. "Fatigue" in patients with multiple sclerosis. Motor pathway conduction and event-related potentials. Arch Neurol 1992; 49:517–524.

13. Rammohan KW, Rosenberg JH, Lynn DJ et al. Efficacy and safety of modefinil (Provigil) for the treatment of fatigue in multiple sclerosis: a two centre phase 2 study. J Neurol Neurosurg Psychiatry 2002; 72:179–183.

14. Peyser JM, Rao SM, LaRocca NG, Kaplan E. Guidelines for neuropsychological research in multiple sclerosis. Arch Neurol 1990; 47:94–97.

15. Prosiegel M, Michael C. Neuropsychology and multiple sclerosis: diagnostic and rehabilitative approaches. J Neurol Sci. 1993; 115:S51–S54.

16. Beatty WW, Goodkin DE, Monson N, Beatty PA. Cognitive disturbances in patients with relapsing remitting multiple sclerosis. Arch Neurol 1989; 46:1113–1119.

17. Comi G, Filippi M, Martinelli V, et al. Brain magnetic resonance imaging correlates of cognitive impairment in multiple sclerosis. J Neurol Sci. 1993; 115:S66–S73.

18. Krupp LB, Elkins LE. Fatigue and declines in cognitive functioning in multiple sclerosis. Neurology 2000; 55:934–939.

19. Boringa JB, Lazeron RH, Reuling IE, et al. The brief repeatable bat-

tery of neuropsychological tests: normative values allow application in multiple sclerosis clinical practice. Mult Scler 2001; 7:263–267.

20. Rao SM, Leo GJ, Ellington L, et al. Cognitive dysfunction in multiple sclerosis. II. Impact on employment and social functioning. Neurology 1991; 41:692–696.

21. Camp SJ, Stevenson VL, Thompson AJ, et al. Cognitive function in primary progressive and transitional progressive multiple sclerosis: a controlled study with MRI correlates. Brain 1999; 122:1341–1348.

22. Clark CM, James G, Li D, et al. Ventricular size, cognitive function and depression in patients with multiple sclerosis. Can J Neurol Sci. 1992; 19:352–356.

23. Moriarty DM, Blackshaw AJ, Talbot PR, et al. Memory dysfunction in multiple sclerosis corresponds to juxtacortical lesion load on fast fluid-attenuated inversion-recovery MR images. Am J Neuroradiol 1999; 20:1956–1962.

24. Rao SM, Leo GJ, Haughton VM, et al. Correlation of magnetic resonance imaging with neuropsychological testing in multiple sclerosis. Neurology 1989; 39:161–166.

25. Rovaris M, Filippi M, Falautano M, et al. Relation between MR abnormalities and patterns of cognitive impairment in multiple sclerosis. Neurology. 1998; 50:1601–1608.

26. Rovaris M, Filippi M, Minicucci L, et al. Cortical/subcortical disease burden and cognitive impairment in patients with multiple sclerosis. Am J Neuroradiol 2000; 21:402–408.

27. Sperling RA, Guttmann CR, Hohol MJ, et al. Regional magnetic resonance imaging lesion burden and cognitive function in multiple sclerosis: a longitudinal study. Arch Neurol 2001; 58:115–121.

28. Medaglini S, Locatelli T, Comi G. ERPs in multiple sclerosis. Ital J Neurol Sci 1998; 19:S408–S412.

29. Plohmann AM, Kappos L, Ammann W, et al. Computer assisted retraining of attentional impairments in patients with multiple sclerosis. J Neurol Neurosurg Psychiatry 1998; 64:455–462.

30. Fischer JS, Priore RL, Jacobs LD, et al. Neuropsychological effects of interferon β-1a in relapsing multiple sclerosis. Multiple Sclerosis Collaborative Research Group. Ann Neurol 2000; 48:885–892.

31. Foong J, Rozewicz L, Quaghebeur G, et al. Neuropsychological deficits in multiple sclerosis after acute relapse. J Neurol Neurosurg Psychiatry 1998; 64:529–532.

32. Giberti L, Croce R, Neri S. Multiple sclerosis and psychiatric disturbances: clinical aspects and a review of the literature. Ital J Neurol Sci 1996; 17:189–191.

33. Rodgers J, Bland R. Psychiatric manifestations of multiple sclerosis: a review. Can J Psychiatry 1996; 41:441–445.

34. Sadovnick AD, Remick RA, Allen J, et al. Depression and multiple sclerosis. Neurology 1996; 46:628–632.

35. Fassbender K, Schmidt R, Mossner R, et al. Mood disorders and dysfunction of the hypothalamic–pituitary–adrenal axis in multiple sclerosis: association with cerebral inflammation. Arch Neurol 1998; 55:66–72.

36. Mohr DC, Goodkin DE, Islar J, et al. Treatment of depression is associated with suppression of nonspecific and antigen-specific T(H)1 responses in multiple sclerosis. Arch Neurol 2001; 58:1081–1086.

37. Mohr DC, Goodkin DE, Likosky W, et al. Treatment of depression improves adherence to interferon β-1b therapy for multiple sclerosis. Arch Neurol 1997; 54:531–533.

38. Neilley LK, Goodin DS, Goodkin DE, Hauser SL. Side effect profile of interferon β-1b in MS: results of an open label trial. Neurology 1996; 46:552–554.

39. Walther EU, Hohlfeld R. Multiple sclerosis: side effects of interferon β therapy and their management. Neurology 1999; 53:1622–1627.

40. Levic ZM, Dujmovic I, Pekmezovic T, et al. Prognostic factors for survival in multiple sclerosis. Mult Scler 1999; 5:171–178.

41. Young RR, Emre M, Nance P, et al. Current issues in spasticity management. Neurologist 1997; 3: 261–275.

42. Bramanti P, Sessa E, Rifici C, et al. Enhanced spasticity in primary progressive MS patients treated with interferon β-1b. Neurology 1998; 51:1720–1723.

43. Ashworth B. Preliminary trial of carisoprodal in multiple sclerosis. Practitioner 1964; 192:540–542.

44. Kita M Goodkin DE. Drugs used to treat spasticity. Drugs 2000; 59:487–495.

45. Wagstaff AJ, Bryson HM. Tizanidine. A review of its pharmacology, clinical efficacy and tolerability in the management of spasticity associated with cerebral and spinal disorders. Drugs 1997; 53:435–452.

46. Mueller ME, Gruenthal M, Olson WL, Olson WH. Gabapentin for relief of upper motor neuron symptoms in multiple sclerosis. Arch Phys Med Rehabil 1997; 78:521–524.

47. Hyman N, Barnes M, Bhakta B, et al. Botulinum toxin (Dysport) treatment of hip adductor spasticity in multiple sclerosis: a prospective, randomised, double blind, placebo controlled, dose ranging study. J Neurol Neurosurg Psychiatry 2000; 68:707–712.

48. Smyth MD, Peacock WJ. The surgical treatment of spasticity. Muscle Nerve 2000; 23:153–163.

49. Paty DW, Noseworthy JH, Ebers GC. Diagnosis of multiple sclerosis. In: Paty DW, Ebers GC, eds. *Multiple Sclerosis*, Philadelphia; F.A. Davis Company; 1998:73.

50. Brisman R. Gamma knife radiosurgery for primary management for trigeminal neuralgia. J Neurosurg 2000; 93:S159–S161.

51. Tüzün E, Akman-Demir G, Eraksoy M. Paroxysmal attacks in multiple sclerosis. Mult Scler 2001; 7:402–404.

52. Alusi SH, Worthington J, Glickman S, Bain PG. A study of tremor in multiple sclerosis. Brain 2001; 124:720–730.

53. Litwiller SE, Frohman EM, Zimmern PE. Multiple sclerosis and the urologist. J Urol 1999; 161:743–757.

54. Andrews KL, Husmann DA. Bladder dysfunction and management in multiple sclerosis. Mayo Clin Proc 1997; 72:1176–1183.

55. Valiquette G, Herbert J, Maede-D'Alisera P. Desmopressin in the management of nocturia in patients with multiple sclerosis. A double-blind, crossover trial. Arch Neurol 1996; 53:1270–1275.

56. Multiple Sclerosis Council For Clinical Pratcie Guidelines Urinary Dysfunction and Multiple Sclerosis. Evidence-Based Management Strategies for Urinary Dysfunction in Multiple Sclerosis. Paralyzed Veterans of America 1999; Washington DC.

57. Barak Y, Achiron A, Elizur A, et al. Sexual dysfunction in relapsing-remitting multiple sclerosis: magnetic resonance imaging, clinical, and psychological correlates. J Psychiatry Neurosci 1996; 21:255–258.

58. Mattson D, Petrie M, Srivastava DK, McDermott M. Multiple sclerosis. Sexual dysfunction and its response to medications. Arch Neurol 1995; 52:862–868.

59. Betts CD, Jones SJ, Fowler CG, Fowler CJ. Erectile dysfunction in multiple sclerosis: associated neurologic deficits and treatment of the condition. Brain 1994; 117:1303–1310.

60. Ghezzi A, Malvestii GM, Baldini S, Zaffaroni S, Zibetti A. Erectile impotence in multiple sclerosis: a neurophysiologic study. J Neurol 1994; 242:123–126.

61. Kirkeby HJ, Poulsen EU, Derup J. Erectile dysfunction in multiple sclerosis. Neurology 1988; 38: 1366–1374.

62. Boolell M, Gepi-Attee S, Gingell JC, Allen MJ. Sildenafil, a novel effective oral therapy for male erectile dysfunction. Br J Urol 1996; 78:257–261.

63. Macdonell RA, Dewey HM. Neurological disability and neurological rehabilitation. *Med J. Aust* 2001; 174:653–658.

64. Petajan JH, White AT. Recommendations for physical activity in patient's with multiple sclerosis. Sports Med 1999; 27:179–191.

Index

Page numbers in bold indicate illustrations; those in italics, tables.